PAIN ERASURE

Bonnie Prudden

PAIN ERASURE:

The Bonnie Prudden Way

By BONNIE PRUDDEN

FOREWORD AND AFTERWORD BY DR. DESMOND TIVY
DRAWINGS BY TERENCE COYLE
PHOTOGRAPHS BY STEPHEN HAWKINS

M. EVANS AND COMPANY, INC. / NEW YORK

Anatomical drawings by Terence Coyle, Lecturer on Anatomy, National Academy of Design and Art Students League of New York and author of *Anatomy Lessons from the Great Masters* and *Albinus on Anatomy*.

In the section "Prevalence of Arthritis by Occupation" in Chapter 6, the list of types of workers has been adapted from *Arthritis* by William Kitay. Copyright © 1977 by William Kitay. Reprint by permission of Monarch Press, a Simon & Schuster division of Gulf & Western Corporation.

M. Evans and Company, Inc.
216 East 49th Street
New York, New York 10017

Library of Congress Cataloging-in-Publication Data

Prudden, Bonnie, 1914–
    Pain Erasure
    Bibliography: p.
    Includes index.
    1. Pain—Prevention. 2. Pain—Treatment. 3. Massage. I.
    Title. [DNLM: 1. Pain—Therapy—Popular works. 2. Exercise
    therapy—Popular works. WL704 P971p]
RB127.P78   616'.0472   80-20688

ISBN 0-87131-983-7

10   9   8   7   6   5   4   3   2   1

This book is dedicated to
DR. JANET TRAVELL

Dr. Travell is many things—doctor, teacher, author, and medical sleuth. It was she who pioneered the work on trigger point injection therapy. It was she who drew the first maps of trigger points and noted that they referred pain to distant places.

It was Dr. Travell's work and her teaching that made the discovery of myotherapy possible. *Thank you,* Dr. Travell.

Pain, not death, is the enemy of mankind. And when you have finished this book, you won't have to be afraid of pain anymore.

BONNIE PRUDDEN

Contents

Acknowledgments

No man (or woman either) is an island, and those of you who get rid of your pain because of this book owe a lot of people a thank you. First, there are the myotherapists who have stood hour after hour working on the muscles of people in pain. Myotherapy isn't anything like plugging in an electric appliance; it requires energy and caring. It can be exhausting. Then there are the people who trusted their pain to a "new" idea. That the success rate is so phenomenal is due in large part to the fact that they persevered with the programs designed for them. Then there is my friend Dr. Desmond Tivy who said over and over in his precise British manner, "Yes, I think you've got something there. . . . Do keep on with it."

During the gestation period needed for this book, the institute staff assumed a great deal of work not really their responsibility; they made sacrifices and labored long hours, and cheerfully at that. My friend Joe Vergara organized mountains of material and brought order out of chaos.

While there would have been no book had it not been for the encouragement and reassurance of Dr. Tivy, there would have been no author but for the quick thinking of Lori Drummond, who once saved my life. But above all, you and I need to thank Enid "Beanie" Whittaker who has worked with this book every inch of the way—and that's a long way, almost five years. She has researched and re-researched, checked and re-checked. She and her husband, Donald Whittaker, and Lori did all the experimental myotherapy on my hip before and after my operation. My nurse, Dee Winslow, also a myotherapist and who figures in the section How to Survive a Hospital, deserves a thank you, at least from me, because nurses, not doctors, determine what your hospital stay will be like.

Lastly, I thank Judy Vachon, without whom I would not have had the courage or know-how to start a school. Six months from now we will graduate our first major group of myotherapists, people you can count on if you hurt.

Note to the Reader

If you like to read long words
If you like to read foreign words
If you like Latin words . . . and medical words
      or strange words,
        enjoy the names of muscles . . .
All that is here for you.
If you like to look at maps
If you like to use maps
If you like to know where you are most of the time . . .
Interesting maps are here for you.
                  BUT
If you don't want to be bothered
with any of that, you just want to be
painfree . . .
JUST LOOK AT THE PICTURES . . . THAT'S ALL HERE,
TOO.

Foreword

IN PRAISE OF BONNIE PRUDDEN

by Dr. Desmond R. Tivy

Bonnie Prudden is a quite remarkable person. Her name is known throughout the United States, by way of her books and her radio and television classes, as that of an ardent and expert proponent of exercise and exercises as a way to physical fitness, efficiency, and health. For some this might have been fame and achievement enough.

Not content with this, however, she has devoted several years to trying to answer a question that has intrigued and plagued her for long, namely: why do so many people hurt in so many odd places that don't seem convincingly explicable by current anatomical and physiological mechanisms, and that don't seem to be predictably relieved by standard medical and physiotherapeutic methods; and what can be done to improve the situation? That's one helluva big question, in reality many questions rolled into one.

The question originated in her observations of her own arthritic hips, which produced strange pains in strange places, with variations in intensity that were not truly consistent with the inexorable progress of the hip degeneration; and in her observations of the response or lack of response of her pains to both standard medical and experimental treatments; and in her observations of similar experiences in those who could not comply with her exercise programs because of pain.

Her answer to the problem developed out of her work with two pioneer doctors in the field, Hans Kraus and Janet Travell, and her studies of the anatomy of muscles and standard and experimental physiotherapy. She noted their successes and the problems they encountered, their lack of general acceptance, and the reasons behind such. Much that she noted and discovered was naturally serendipitous, since most discoveries are. What came out of all this was a collation of mostly non-original ideas, in an original way, which is the mark of brilliance. Such an achievement requires hard concentrated work (and thus energy), and keen powers of observation together with an open mind (and thus intelligence), as well as great integrity (and thus honesty). Bonnie Prudden exhibits these qualities above all. Add to this, humor and flair, and you have what it takes to do what she has done. Unfortunately she also happens to have a superlative bedside manner. I say "unfortunately," though I suppose she would not have cared enough to do what she has done if she had not possessed it. What is unfortunate is that her critics have attributed and will attribute her therapeutic successes to faith, and the fact that "she cares."

I would ask such critics to examine the evidence more closely. Almost *any* therapy, this included, works *better* when therapist and patient have confidence in it. But myotherapy seems also to work quite well when therapist or patient or both show no such confidence, provided always that the indication to use it happens to be present, and the same can be said about penicillin. If not Faith, then what of Hope? Whenever penicillin does not have the ability to work, I do not find that *hoping* it will work, will *make* it work any more often than coincidence would allow; the same applies to myotherapy. Many doctors with excellent bedside manners and who care deeply seem unable to relieve some of the types of pain on which myotherapy works, so charm alone seems insufficient: all pain is worsened by lack of patient confidence (i.e., fear), so the beginning of pain relief by a therapist will promote confidence and further pain relief. It certainly seems to help to discover that your therapist is competent; and a good bedside manner, to quote Bonnie, "sure doesn't do any harm!" She has trained quite a few myotherapists now. Their results seem as good as hers, and their bedside manners are also good. But it seems it is their technique that is crucial to the results.

I will not attempt to define myotherapy or the conditions on which it may be tried, since this is to be found in the text. But I can say that I have had several years to study her methods and results on several hundreds of patients: I am convinced that both are valid. I obviously cannot confirm all that she claims, because

I was not "there" to do it. However, I can testify that, study her as you will, her methods and results are, in general, remarkable, largely predictable, and safe. Bonnie Prudden has here presented her admittedly tentative results, in a not very tentative way, so that the world may find out for itself, by independent testing, how sound such testimony is.

For those interested enough to pursue the study of myotherapy further, I have expounded at some length in an Afterword, on various central and peripheral issues of relevance. It may help others to assess her competence as a therapist, and my competence as a judge, the better. It might possibly discourage the overadventurous. And it may possibly encourage some fearful souls, who, afraid of doing harm, end up never trying anything new.

Most People Don't Have to Suffer Pain

Most people don't have to suffer pain. Most pain can be erased by what you are about to learn. To believe this hopeful news all you need do is follow directions.

This book is designed to help people who hurt or who have friends, relatives or teammates who hurt.

Everything presented here has been tried over and over again and it all does work, but you won't really know that until you have tried it yourself. Relief from all kinds of pain can be had, often within minutes. To do this requires no special training, no special diet, no medicines at all. It does require that the pain be muscular, but then most pain is muscular pain anyway.

The technique for erasing pain is called myotherapy, and it is remarkable. The list of successes grows daily and takes in more and more conditions causing pain. Not only does the therapy help the pain you have now, but it prevents its recurrence as well. The details and how-to are covered in the chapters that follow. For now, here is a quick explanation of how it works.

Myotherapy involves an entity known in medical circles as a trigger point. Just what a trigger point is, is debatable. That it exists is not. Trigger points are found in muscles that have been "insulted," which in medicalese means "damaged," and damage can begin even before birth. It seems that trigger points can lie quiet in muscles, often for years, but when the climate is right, and such a climate usually involves physical and emotional stress, they seem to light up. When that happens, the muscles in which they reside tighten. If those muscles are in your neck, you wake with your head at a painful angle. If they are in your back you join the backache crowd. If it is in the muscles under your scalp, you develop headaches. After a while the trigger point may calm down, the muscles relax, and you think you are fine. You aren't; you are merely relieved for a while. The trigger point is still there and will light up again when your stress level is raised. No one has ever seen a trigger point, and when biopsies are performed on painful muscles, no trigger points are found. Speculation of course ranges all over the lot, but that is not our concern. Detriggering the trigger point is—and that we can do. Now.

Fran Cormier's mother was in her late sixties and had so much back pain that she could no longer manage in her little Florida home. All the tests had been done and all available treatments and medications had been tried. As a last resort she was to be fitted with a brace. She would have to sell her little place and move back north to live with her daughter. The guest room had already been equipped with a hospital bed and a walker when Fran called to ask if we could see her mother. It was just a small glimmer of hope, she said, but her mother wanted to try myotherapy.

Fran brought her mother to us, and we worked with her for one hour. The charming little woman felt so good when she left that she forgot her cane. Fran and her daughter Leslie learned how to work with their getting-spryer-every-day guest. The walker is now used for a towel rack and the hospital bed went back where it came from. Fran's mother went back, too, to Florida. She sold her house there, bought a condominium, and gives weekly exercise classes in the community room for her neighbors.

She has pain once in a while, at which point she hops a plane for Connecticut where she gets "detriggered," has a nice visit with her family, and then hops a plane back down again. A far cry from what happens when most pain-filled "elderlies" pay their annual duty visit to their children in the north.

· Mark, at the other end of the age scale, was only 23. He had been so smashed up in a car accident that for months before he came to us all he could move was his left thumb. We worked with him once a week for six months, and his father did some work on him every day. Mark is now able to walk from the car to our treatment room. He rides a tandem bike with his dad and drives the car. His speech improves all the time, as do his strength and coordination. Mark's dad bet a hundred dollars (to go to the Red Cross) that on a given day the boy would swim the length of the pool. We were all rooting for him and were sure he'd make it. When the phone call came through with the news, we learned he had swum *six* lengths.

To find out if untrained people could find and erase trigger points, we set up a study with first graders. An anatomy text was designed for their comprehension level. These six-year-olds learned the names of muscles in no time at all, and with the help of "Muscle Man" and "Mr. Bones" drawn life-size on cardboard, could tell which on the one moved what on the other. The class learned the myotherapy technique quickly, and there wasn't an untreated case of growing pains in the group. If the teacher didn't erase the pains, the little kids did. When their classmate Carl broke his leg, they studied fractures. When the leg came out of the cast, they predicted where there would be trigger points—and that's exactly where they found them.

WHAT MYOTHERAPY IS, ITS MEDICAL ORIGINS, AND HOW IT ERASES PAIN

For myotherapy to be born, I had to know three of the many pioneering contributors. In the order in which I met them, they are Dr. Hans Kraus, Dr. Janet Travell, and Dr. Desmond Tivy.

Dr. Kraus's contribution came 42 years ago. It happened this way. I was mountain climbing with friends and woke the second morning with a very painful stiff neck. I'd had them off and on for years, ever since a fall from a bucking horse. Dr. Kraus, a member of the party, looked at my lopsided head and allowed that I wouldn't be much good on a climb in my condition. He placed a thumb on the back of my neck and pressed so hard my knees buckled. That didn't stop him; he knew what he was doing. He meant to squash that knot whatever it took. Climbers are fanatics and nothing must get in the way of a climb. I was hard put not to cry, but when he let up, my head was on straight. There was no pain at all. Off we went for a magnificent climb.

Meanwhile, Dr. Travell had pioneered a medical discipline called trigger point injection therapy. In this therapy, the doctor usually probes with a finger until a tender spot, indicating the presence of a trigger point, is found. The spot is then in-

3

jected with a solution, usually saline and procaine. The doctors tell you the injections don't hurt, but that's because they are on the painless end of the needle. Dr. Travell follows her injections with a gentle passive stretch, usually aided by the coolant spray Fluori-Methane. Other doctors use electrical stimulation and/or analgesics. While myotherapy and trigger point injection therapy have elements in common, there is one major difference. Myotherapy involves no injections whatsoever.

It was 1976 before all the pieces of the myotherapy puzzle finally fell into place. Enter Dr. Tivy.

For many years I had been working with medically referred patients, providing them with corrective exercises after operations or trigger point injection therapy. At the time, Dr. Tivy and I had developed a comfortable working arrangement, dealing mostly with back patients with whom I would work after Dr. Tivy had injected their trigger points. Or when someone came to me first, through my classes, I would send him or her on to Dr. Tivy. Then after injection the patient would come back to me for correctives. The patients showed improvement, and I felt we were doing a good service.

One morning a woman arrived with her head all lopsided. She had a very painful stiff neck. By this time, I'd established the practice of finding the trigger points myself, circling them in ink, and then shipping the patient over to Dr. Tivy for injection. As I was probing around in the muscles at the back of her neck I found what I was looking for, a very tender spot—a trigger point. I'll never know exactly what I did, perhaps press a little harder or hold a little longer than was my custom, but, "Yikes! That was awful!" said the woman, turning to me with her head now held straight. The surprise on her face mirrored the surprise on mine. Was it possible that the slight pressure I had exerted on the patient's trigger point had relieved her stiff neck? Without benefit of an injection? I was determined to find out.

My next appointment was with a woman who had a painful tennis elbow. Ordinarily I would have tried to improve the range of the joint with resistance exercises. This time I didn't. I warned her that trigger points are very tender and I sought them as though she were being mapped for injection. But instead of marking the arm I held the trigger point. It was painful. Instead of settling for one trigger point I probed up and down the entire arm, pressing trigger points as I found them. In about 15 minutes there was no pain, and both elbow and shoulder had full range of movement. I really was onto something important!

As soon as the patient left, I raced for the phone and called Washington to tell Dr. Travell about my exciting discovery.

She asked one question, "How long did you hold the pressure?"

"About four seconds."

"May not be long enough. Try longer."

I tried holding the pressure for fifteen seconds and worked back to seven. Seven seems about right for most trigger points except for those in the face and head. You can usually get the same good results with those in four or five seconds.

In my Myotherapy Institute, we worked at first mainly with backs. Instead of taking weeks to get rid of pain with exercise and injections, it was taking only a few sessions, often only one. Arm pain, shoulder and neck pain, all surrendered. We even had several stroke patients who were being given stretch and strengthening exercises. Two of them had severely contracted arm muscles. Soon they too were free of pain and their limbs of contracture.

We were getting fine results erasing pains caused by hurt muscles. But what about headaches? Do they involve muscles? Can myotherapy help headaches? I found out the day I happened to visit Dr. Tivy.

"I've got a ten-year-old girl with migraine in my office. Would you look at her," said Dr. Tivy.

The little girl had had the headache for several days. "Always has headaches," was offered by the distraught mother.

"When did she fall off her horse?" I asked. (Little girls fall off horses, little boys out of trees.)

"She always falls off her horse, and she fell off the swing so often I had her father take it down."

I started my search for trigger points on the little girl's neck and continued over the scalp, down the shoulders, and right into the seat muscles. Trigger points were everywhere, but in half an hour the pain was gone. Next day I got a strange call from her mother.

"What do I do with her now?"

I asked if the headache was back. "No."

"Well, then, don't do anything. She'll probably be fine

unless she falls off her horse again, and then the same pain with the same trigger points may come back. If they do, we'll repeat the treatment."

The girl was back in a month. Her horse had tossed its head back against her head—hard. It took an hour to clear her head, neck, and shoulder muscles—and teach the mother how to do it for her. That kid was going to need an on-the-site maintenance crew.

And that's how we came to insist that anyone coming to us from a distance bring a friend or relative we can instruct. That gives the patient two benefits: a way to get rid of pain should it recur, plus a feeling of security, since someone near knows how to help.

And now it's your turn. Let's learn how to locate the trigger points for specific pains, how to erase them, and which stretching exercises reinforce the treatment. And then you too will be able to rid yourself and those close to you of pain.

To Erase Pain, Erase 2. Trigger Points

Before we talk about erasing pain let us discuss some facts about pain.

For our purposes there are two kinds of pain, chronic and acute. Acute pain is understandable, is valuable, and has a foreseeable end. Most of us would not have survived childhood without it, for acute pain is a warning pain. It is acute pain that tells you that the cavity your tongue has been investigating for a month is now past ignoring. Acute pain insists that you snatch your hand off the hot stove or stop sawing away on the lemon because your finger is in the way. Acute pain also announces some form of pathology. Appendicitis is a good example, as is a fractured ankle. Whether the cause is cutting, burning, fracturing, or disease, the pain suggests immediate medical intervention for an obvious cause which even the sufferer can understand. That part is most important to peace of mind—which is often a factor in healing—as is this fact: There is usually a time limit on acute pain. Bad as it may be, it will not last forever. Whether you yell, groan, or grin and bear it; whether you take a painkiller or refuse such help; whether you have a cut that will heal in one week or a fracture requiring six—you know what you have and that there will be an end to it.

Chronic pain is very different.

Anatomic pathology is rarely attached to chronic pain. It isn't the same at all as a nice clear-cut case of strep throat.

While acute pain is a warning, chronic pain may or may not have an observable cause. Or the observable cause, say, back strain after lifting a piano, is not the real cause at all, but

7

merely a triggering mechanism for an underlying cause, trigger points.

Most chronic pain is caused by a condition in the muscles. Disease is responsible for some of it, but just plain living is the cause of far more.

Painkillers Don't Kill Pain

In addition to our ignorance about pain, what causes it, and what can be done about it, there is ignorance too about the painkillers we gobble in incredible quantities. Painkillers probably raise pain thresholds so you are not aware of the pain, but it keeps on pulsing just the same.

We begin our story with two words: trigger points.

WHAT A TRIGGER POINT IS AND HOW IT FUNCTIONS

We probably shouldn't call this section "What a Trigger Point Is . . ." since we don't know exactly, but we do know it is a highly irritable spot in a muscle and contributes critically to pain. Whether it is chemical, electrical, or right out of Pandora's box will one day be determined by research, but for now, please just accept it as something very real with which we must deal.

Trigger points are laid down in muscles all through life. Any of a number of things—a fall, blow, knock, strain, or sprain, for example—can insult the muscles. Opportunities present themselves constantly.

The Spasm-Pain-Spasm Cycle

A trigger point lies quiet in a muscle until the physical and emotional climate is right, and then it "fires." Its firing throws the muscle into spasm. This causes pain, and the autonomic nervous system comes complete with plans for handling pain. It sends more spasm to the affected area to protect it against whatever is threatening.

When the spasm sent by the nervous system reaches the designated area, it further tightens the spasm already present. That hurts! Another pain message shoots back to headquarters predictably followed by yet more spasm. This phenomenon is called "splinting." We now have a spasm-pain-spasm cycle in effect, and until it is broken the pain will continue unabated, and as the pain continues, so will the splinting. This shortens the muscles and holds them in a foreshortened condition, which not only causes pain but interferes with function, posture, and balance. If the cycle is maintained long enough, the muscles may remain permanently shortened.

There are numerous ways to break the spasm-pain-spasm cycle—analgesics, such as aspirin, or something stronger, such as codeine, for example. Counterirritants, such as liniment, are a classic remedy. Heat, both moist and dry, is tried, as are cold, rest, injections, and so on. When one of these works, the sufferer is apt to think, "Thank goodness that's over." But it isn't over. The trigger point has simply backed off to await another day—and that day will inevitably come.

Satellite Trigger Points

If the spasm-pain-spasm episode was serious, the original trigger point may have added to itself in the form of satellite trigger points, which were laid down in the same and neighboring muscles when those muscles were thrown into fiber-tearing spasm. They do not seem to possess the same potential for referring pain to other muscles as do the key, or matrix, trigger points, but they do seem to have the ability to rekindle the fires in the matrix trigger points. It is knowledge about and the handling of these satellites that is the key to the startling success of myotherapy.

THE MAJOR CAUSES OF TRIGGER POINTS

Birth

Being born often produces the first batch of trigger points. The baby may arrive all bruised and battered, or with its poor little head as pointy as a gnome's. Nobody is too concerned. After all, it happens all the time. (Read LeBoyer's *Birth Without Violence* and you'll see there is a way to minimize such distress.)

In a few weeks the baby's bruises will fade. To all eyes, except those of a myotherapist who has worked with birth-damaged babies, all is well. The trigger points established may lie dormant for months, or even years, but nursing or teething may provide just the triggering mechanism needed to bring them to

9

life. Then the baby and its parents will pay the price of ignorance—weeks of screaming. It will probably be called colic, but colic is often only the result of screaming for hours on end and swallowing air all the while. The real cause may well be a banging, pounding headache. (See under The Baby Who Arrived in a Hurry, in Chapter 8.)

Accidents

A minor fall off a curb, at the ice rink, or on a ski slope that bruises a tailbone (coccyx) will soon be forgotten. No one will connect it with low back pain, "sciatica," hemorrhoids, and certainly never with frigidity or impotence that strikes years later. However, check the floor of the pelvis (see Appendix 1, Plate 19), and you will understand how easily trigger points anywhere in those muscles could affect a number of important functions.

The auto accident that very nearly totals both car and driver is rightly expected to have some long-term effects. But the skid into a tree that merely knocks out a headlight and gives the driver a stiff neck can hardly be considered a contributing factor when, ten years later, the driver exhibits symptoms of "cervical arthritis" (a pain in the neck).

No accident is trivial. All accidents have the potential for laying down trigger points. They may lie hidden for years only to reappear when the time is ripe.

Sports

In the name of good, clean sport, we do ourselves a lot of damage. Don't blame sport. We would be poverty stricken without it. No. We do harm because of ignorance. We don't know how to prevent injury. Half the time we don't even know we are injured. Then when the injury becomes so obvious we can't overlook it, we haven't a notion as to what to do about it.

The sport called jogging puts trigger points in the leg muscles. These often cause muscle cramps in the legs and lead to a condition called shinsplints. When trigger points in the leg muscles "fire," the muscles in spasm pull on the knee joint, which begins to ache. Over a million joggers in the last year have reported knee injuries. Usually the aching knee is then taped. Or it may be soaked in a whirlpool bath, or rubbed with liniment. It may be fitted with an elastic knee bandage or even one fitted with a metal brace. In any case the trigger points go right on firing and the spasm-pain-spasm cycle remains very much in effect, causing pain and even brand new trigger points which will add their voices to the clamor.

Occupation

Each job, like each sport, has its own pattern of trigger points. The shape of that pattern depends on the way the body is used, underused, or overused during work. Operating a jack-hammer all day, like playing football, will jar just about everything. The horse jockey gets it in the neck, upper back, and right leg. The disc jockey, sitting all day lifting nothing heavier than a record, gets it in the back, shoulders, and both legs. We expect the moving man to get backaches. But executives get them too. And the occupation "only a housewife" is as fraught with peril as that of a stunt driver.

Disease

Rheumatoid arthritis and multiple sclerosis are typical of diseases that generate trigger points. Strokes too lay them down. Even a high fever will do it, as will diseased organs and joints.

Trigger points get into the act when arthritis is active. Like multiple sclerosis, the pain of arthritis comes and goes. When it's out of town, called remission, the sufferer can be without pain or nearly so. That, incidentally, is the time to embrace a strong exercise program. It is essential that muscles be kept flexible and that all joints be capable of moving through the full range of motion. Then when the disease strikes again the body is prepared to do battle.

Even in cases so extreme that surgery is performed, pain may persist. Consider a patient with disc disease who must undergo an operation. The disc, badly ruptured and pressing on a nerve, is removed. The bones fuse properly, there is no infection, and the patient has come through with flying colors—except that the pain is as bad as before. The surgeon is stymied. The family doctor is stymied. What went wrong? What went wrong was that the disc disease was cleared up, but the trigger points remained. Indeed, the operation may even have produced a few new trigger points of its own. The surgeon got rid of the disease. Myotherapy will get rid of the pain.

11

HOW A STRESSFUL CLIMATE TRIGGERS PAIN

Let's recap quickly. A trigger point is laid down when a muscle is insulted. It lies doggo until the "climate" is right and then something sets it off. What sort of climate is right, and what kind of something will activate a trigger point?

Climate has to do with stress. Stress can be pleasant, but usually the climate for pain is unpleasant. No matter what lays down trigger points, trauma or disease, or when they are laid down, the emotional stress which is a part of living plays a major role in chronic pain. Here is an example.

Trigger Points + Stress + Triggering Mechanism = Chronic Pain

A young patient had a skiing accident and smashed her pelvis. Many muscles were badly mistreated. Despite doomsday predictions—"You'll always walk with a limp," "You'll never have children,"—she recovered and went on to do all the things she'd always wanted to do and happily thumbed her nose at the doctors.

Unhappily, as time went on her marriage began to deteriorate. Now this young woman had been brought up when people believed in the adage, "You made your bed, now lie in it." In those days it didn't matter if there were toads or snakes in that bed or that it was on fire or at the bottom of a well; you were expected to stay and make the best of it. The climate in her home became more and more tense. And along with the climate, every one of her muscles was tensing and stiffening, some to the point of spasm.

For months her back had been aching as she went about her daily chores. One night after a particularly trying afternoon she carried little Number Two Daughter into the bathroom. As she leaned over to set the sleepy child on the potty, something went *crack*. Down she went, baby and all. Her back had gone into spasm. The trigger points laid down seven years before— and silent until her life began to heat up—had struck. The stressful emotional climate surrounded her. The triggering mechanism was the strain caused by the awkward forward reach required to seat the child.

SOME BY-PRODUCTS OF PAIN

As if pain itself weren't making life hard enough, it is often accompanied by other difficulties. Let's look at some of pain's by-products.

Employment Climate in Business—Often Deadly

The climate that surrounds business people can be destructive, indeed. Consider. You are caught up in the frantic climb up the corporate ladder. Just as the prize seems within reach, you are suddenly out of a job. Corporations seem to act that way often. They give their middle management people bright, young apprentices. Then one day there's a shakeup and the apprentices have the jobs and the bosses are out job hunting.

Hanging on during change is another grinding experience. Did you ever wonder what happened to the mills that produced cotton stockings, cotton underwear, and cotton shirts? And the factories that bent wire into bobby pins? And the Momma-Poppa shops when supers took over? A lot of grinding down has been going on. There are always winners and losers. Losing can create a miserable emotional climate.

Pain and Fatigue. The person who has pain for a bedfellow sleeps badly and often awakens more tired than the night before. One of the surest signs that myotherapy is doing its job is a good night's sleep.

If people didn't hurt they would have the energy and strength to bounce back from strain and disappointment. They could start out all over again. I've started over again so many times I feel like a race horse that is perpetually at the starting gate. Most people can manage their lives well enough if they are rested and free from pain.

Pain and Irritation. Bosses who have shoulder and neck pains are hard to live with. Employees who have to leave early with headaches or who call in sick with backaches are no bargain either. Everyone suffers—those who have the pain and those who have to put up with people who have pain.

Pain and Self-Image. If you hurt, there is strain in your face. A backache or hip pain interferes with your balance. You feel unsure of yourself. Shoulder pain can make your back look

13

hunched over and round. And it can make you look old beyond your years. If you hurt, you won't be proud of what you see in a mirror.

Pain and Dependency. If your pain is such that you can't get out of the house, can't drive your car, can't even tie your shoelaces, you may be still alive but you are not living. And soon, someone is going to head you toward a nursing home.

But none of this is inevitable. The answer is simple. Get rid of the pain. And learn how to keep it away from you.

IMPORTANCE OF A HEALTHY CLIMATE IN WARDING OFF PAIN

It is not enough in myotherapy to detrigger the trigger points and relax the muscle with stretching exercises. It is not enough, even if you follow with a regular exercise program geared to improve strength and flexibility and to raise your fitness level. You must always be aware of the powerful effects of your emotional climate and how damaging it can be to muscles when it gets out of hand. You must not only be aware, you must be willing to change it.

If you saw your executive dreams evaporating, your house up for sale, your wife back to teaching, and—unthinkable—your second car being driven by a distant relative, would that be so terrible if you felt strong, healthy, and ready to take on Ali—or the job market? No, it probably wouldn't. And the changes might even be good for everyone, especially you.

We must face the fact that emotional climate plays a star role in chronic pain. First, understand the problem. Second, get rid of the pain. Third, get fit, with plenty of endurance. Then, if the climate of your life is unbearable, change the bed you made or burn it. Make a better bed. And never lie in it more than eight hours out of twenty-four.

14

Techniques Used in Myotherapy 3.

WHY MYOTHERAPY WORKS

After about the two-hundredth successful treatment in my institute, I called Dr. Travell and told her about the results we were obtaining with myotherapy. Then I asked her the question so many others had asked me: "Why does it work?"

Her answer was short and direct. "You are denying the trigger point oxygen."

Now if I deny you oxygen, you will up and die. If I tie a string tightly around the base of your finger so no oxygen can get past, the finger will in time turn black and fall off. Why shouldn't a little spot in a muscle give up its nasty little ghost if I deny it oxygen? Anyway, Dr. Travell says it does.

Ten days from now, or ten years from now, someone may come up with a very complicated set of reasons to explain why trigger points lose their power to cause pain when squashed for seven seconds, but we really don't have time to wait. Too many people hurt right now. Too many wonderful musicians, athletes, and actors are having their careers destroyed, and too many babies are screaming right now. If you have so much as a throb in your little finger, it's too much to ignore while research winds its tortuous way along the trails of knowledge. Myotherapy's help is available right now; let's use it. Time will raise the curtain on the play, but let's get the actresses and actors ready now, by clothing them in beautiful, painfree bodies.

HOW DO YOU GET STARTED?

Only those trained in anatomy can look at a body and immediately see bones and muscles. With practice however, you will soon find yourself getting so good at it you will un-skin everyone you know. But first you need to know what the human anatomy looks like.

The anatomy plates in Appendix 1 at the back of this book will provide you with all you need to know for starters. Constant referral to that section as you work on yourself and your friends and relatives (myotherapy also works for pets) will give you considerable information on the bodies of others and your own. After a time when someone says they have a pain in the arm you will be able to predict where the "pain in the arm" is really coming from and you will know the name of the muscle hiding the culprit trigger point. Knowing the name, address, and MO of a criminal is what the FBI needs to know. You are now in the detective business, too.

What Should You Have on Hand?

You will need tracing paper. This will be used in connection with the trigger point maps you will be making. You will also need four different colored pens, preferably a black one for tracing, a blue one for the first session with your subjects, red for the second, and yellow for the third.

You will also need a table. Almost any sturdy raised surface will do—the kitchen or dining room table, a desk, a workbench, or even a pool table. If your table is four feet long and your subject six, put a pillow over the back of a chair and let him rest his leftover length on that.

You *can* do trigger point work on a cot or firm bed, but it may prove tiring. In an emergency you may even use the floor, but the angles are wrong, which makes the work difficult.

To search out trigger points, you will use your fingers, knuckles and elbows and a Bodo. Fingers and knuckles are fine for smaller jobs, such as those done on the arm and some leg muscles. Knuckles work well in many places, but don't use them on the ribs of babies and older people. Elbows are invaluable in areas where considerable force is required.

Bodos are wooden dowels attached to wooden handles and come in three sizes. We use the smallest on hands and feet.

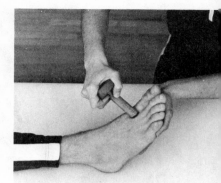

The others are not needed if you have someone at home who can work on you. If you live alone or travel alone, you may need all three. (See the Sources section at the back of this book for information about obtaining Bodos.)

A prime place for a trigger point if you have a long second toe is on top of the instep. (See under The Classic Greek Foot in Chapter 6.) You can reach this with a knuckle if you are limber, but it is virtually impossible to get at the others that invariably team up with it and reside in the underside of the foot. With a Bodo you can. You can also reach those in the back of your neck and shoulders. The gymnast in the illustration here is demonstrating the way to use a Bodo in the seat muscle, the gluteus maximus, which is the favorite residence for trigger points causing most back pain. A sawed-off broom handle will work fairly well in an emergency, but it is the Bodo's handle that gives it control and force.

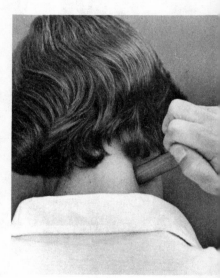

While not absolutely necessary, Fluori-Methane, a coolant spray, certainly speeds the antipain process. You will have to get a prescription from your doctor for the spray. Our first-graders who, praise be, can't get prescriptions, use the corners of ice cubes. They will tell you this works, but with one drawback. "It's messy." One theory (there are several) on the way coolant works is that cold travels along nerve pathways faster than does pain. The spray therefore preempts the communication lines and the autonomic nervous system doesn't get the pain message signaling the need for spasm. It is used while stretching the affected muscle *after* myotherapy has extinguished the trigger points. Sprayed along the painful area, it augments relaxation.

THE TECHNIQUE FOR APPLYING PRESSURE

What you do then, is search out and neutralize trigger points. After finding the first one you move along the muscle at one-inch intervals like a local commuter train stopping at every station from one end of its run to the other. At each station you press down. If you have found a trigger point you hold the pressure for seven seconds. If there is no trigger point you move on to the next station.

Your question about now is probably "But how will I know when I've found one?"

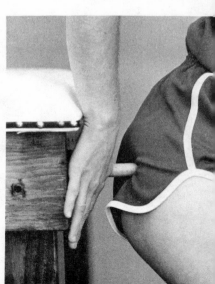

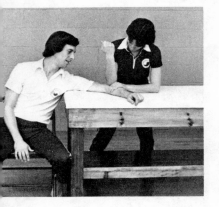

No problem. If you are working on yourself, you will soon be painfully aware of finding one. If you are working on someone else, that person will let you know in no uncertain terms. He or she will holler, groan, grimace, twist, or twitch—and you will know. It is usually best to explain exactly what it is you intend to do and how you plan to go about it. Explain, too, that while trigger points do hurt when unearthed, the object is to extinguish them—not the person on the table.

Before you tackle a real job, you need to know what searching for a trigger point feels like yourself. Now you need a sympathetic friend. Have the friend sit next to a table. Have him or her lay one arm flat, palm down, with the entire length of the arm up to the armpit in contact with the table surface. Place your working elbow (try to use the same one constantly, because with practice, it will develop a "feel") in position just below the elbow joint. Most people have a trigger point there; it is one of the two guiltiest ones in "tennis elbow." Use your other hand to circle your elbow so it cannot slip off. You will find the muscles of the arm numbered according to the order of attack on Plate 17 in Appendix 1.

Press straight down very slowly as though your arm worked hydraulically. If there is tenderness verging on pain, you have found what you are seeking, a trigger point. Hold that pressure for the required seven seconds and then *slowly* release the pressure.

There is one precaution you should take. Assure your friend that what you need is a map, not a hero. He or she gives you that map by telling you where it hurts and how much it hurts. Macho bear-it-in-silence helps no one, least of all the silent sufferer. After you have shown your friend what a trigger point feels like, change places so *you* will know.

Next you will need to know how much pressure to apply. Put your bathroom scale on a table and cover it with a folded bath towel. Press down until the scale registers about 15 to 20 pounds. That would be plenty of pressure for the average arm. If the subject is a child or an elderly person or someone extremely sensitive to pain, of course you use less. You will use more pressure (up to 30 and 40 pounds) on the gluteals in the seat, and less pressure (as little as 6 pounds) on the face. If the painful muscle does not give up spasm, press a little harder. If the subject can't take the pain, use less pressure.

Easy Does It

Keep in mind that you don't have to do the whole job at one time. If you make a good map and follow it, you will know from day to day what you did and where you did it, what you found and where you must go from there.

Remember, there is no need to go for broke with every trigger point. That to my mind, is what happens when the trigger point injections are given. The needle (and it isn't a little needle most of the time) has invaded the body. The doctor's impulse to be thorough is very strong. And since necessary but time-consuming precautions against infection have been taken, the doctor understandably wants to treat every last trigger point his needle can find. You, on the other hand, have no such urgency. With myotherapy you can do a little today and more tomorrow. You can take three minutes during a TV commercial or half an hour before bedtime. If an area is very sensitive, you can "open it up," which means search once over lightly. Then in a few days you can bring more pressure to bear.

Because the muscles have been in spasm a long time— and have had it their own way, so to speak—the first session is always the worst. From then on it usually gets easier, less painful, and even more effective.

At the end of Chapter 7, you will read about massage and learn how to follow up a session with double massage, which is totally relaxing. In addition, you will learn how to use a technique called seeking massage, which can unearth potential trouble spots even when there is no pain. This is an excellent way to *prevent* pain.

HOW TO MAKE A TRIGGER POINT MAP

Myotherapy involves a partnership between the person erasing the trigger points and the subject. If you are acting as your own myotherapist, you are in good hands. Working on someone else, you provide the tools—your fingers, knuckles, and elbow— while the subject provides the information for your in-depth trigger point map.

Once you have selected a painful area to be mapped, the next task is to identify the probable source of the pain and which muscles will be involved, at least primarily. You can do that by

19

looking up the appropriate plate in Appendix 1 and by reading the sections in this book about the area that is hurting, that is, the back, head, arm, leg, or so on. Make a tracing of the plate or plates that shows the muscles you intend to work on. Lay the tracing on the table next to your subject. Then begin your search, *not* according to the most painful spot, for example, the middle of the lower back in lower back pain, but according to the directions provided. (In the case of low back pain you begin in spots 1, 2, and 3 in the gluteals, the seat, as shown in Plate 5.)

When you find a trigger point, press on it and ask your subject what level of pain your pressure is causing. Use a scale of 1 to 10. One, 2, and 3 are mild. Four, 5, and 6 are uncomfortable, 8 and 9 are bad, and 10 is awful. There are always people who will shout, "Twenty-two!" or "Pay dirt!" Others will be very precise. One doctor-mathematician-musician has said softly, "Seven and three quarters . . ." Be sure your subject knows that he or she can say "Stop!" at any time and that you will let up your pressure. Too much pain causes tensing of other muscles, which only defeats the purpose.

Once you begin to make the map, it's helpful to have a second person "scan" for you. A scanner stands by, following your every move, and marking the map accordingly. If when pressure is applied the subject says, "Oh, that's about a two. No real pain, only pressure," the scanner makes a tiny dot on the corresponding spot on the map. That would represent deep water on a sea chart, no shoals there. If, however, it's definitely a tender spot, one of the "Ouch" variety, then an x is entered. If it's one of those variously referred to as dilly!, corker!, or "Oh my God!" then the x is circled.

These marks will be made with the appropriate color pen, as explained earlier: blue for the first session, red for the second, yellow for the third. Because the satellite trigger points (see Chapter 2) are usually wiped out in one or two sessions, they will generally show up only in blue, with an occasional red mark. The matrix, taking longer, can be quite colorful indeed.

Mara is in her late seventies and she came to us three years ago with a "terrible back." It took six sessions to get rid of it, although she was much better after the first one. At the end of summer she went back to her winter home in New Orleans, painfree. She had no more pain for half the winter, then she fell off a lawn chair and it began to creep back. When spring came Mara stopped by for a few weeks on her way to England for her annual visit. She was hurting and terrified that her back would go into spasm while she was far from home . . . and us. We suggested she wear a second pair of underpants for her next sessions, a pair we could draw on. That would give her a "map" she could take along. By the end of the fourth session, we had created a work of art. The matrix points were those with three or more colors, and if any of them referred pain to somewhere else, that information was included with the help of arrows.

Mara went to England feeling very secure, but she did get one backache after a tour of the Lake Country. She put on her colorful underpants and hied herself down to her niece's doctor and said, "I have a backache. Please push with your elbow wherever there are three colors. Hold that pressure for seven seconds." It worked fine and the English doctor asked for a lesson.

The Value of the Map
Besides being useful for such unusual purposes, the trigger point map will provide all kinds of information. These are some suggestions for uses you can put the map to:

1. The marks are a record of trigger points already located and pressed. A glance will prevent your attacking a given area a second time during the session, which might make it sore, or leave a bruise.
2. You will know which trigger points were "awful" the first time, but milder the second time.
3. You will know where the matrix trigger points are, and if the pain should return at some later date, it would save you hunting time. That's where they will be again.
4. You will know where you found the satellites.
5. You will know exactly where the matrix "holdouts" are. These are the ones that are always tender even when the subject no longer is. Those are especially important for the athlete. If he or she has holdouts, they should be checked before any competition lest the trigger point and its incipient spasm burst forth at the height of the game. That could sideline a player for a week, a month, a year, or always.

21

THE END-OF-SESSION STRETCH AND OTHER EXERCISE

After treating three or four trigger points, follow with the appropriate stretching exercises. These are described in the chapter covering the area of the body that you worked on. The stretch exercises are a must both during the myotherapy work and for several days afterward. They play an important part since they re-educate the muscles newly freed of spasm. Next, you will need to set up an exercise program for your subject. Check with the exercise and fitness chapter and the Appendixes having to do with occupations and sports so you will be able to put together a program that fits the subject's life style.

Importance of the Fitness Test

You should take (or administer) the Kraus-Weber Fitness Test in Chapter 10. That will tell you whether you or your subject have any deficiencies in the key posture muscles—the abdominals, the back, the psoas (I'll bet that's one you didn't know you had), and the hamstrings (the tendons in the back of the legs). It is sometimes hard to determine which comes first, the inadequate musculature, which causes trigger points, or the trigger points, which cause inadequate musculature. Proper exercises can correct weaknesses and help avoid pain resulting from poor muscle tone.

KNOW YOUR SUBJECT'S HISTORY

What has happened over the years to cause the pain you, your friend, or your relative suffers? Somewhere, back there among the shadows, there is a reason. The first book I wrote on this subject was called *Dolor Fallax, The Elusive Pain*. It is elusive because its origins are elusive. Once you know what started the whole thing, the pain is no longer elusive but very understandable. Let me show you.

Dr. Tivy sent me a woman who had had abdominal pain for 35 years. Everything possible had been tried, except surgery. She refused that on the grounds that she didn't want to get a pain to find a pain. The pain she had she knew she could stand, if just barely. I asked her the following questions, which you should ask your patient.

Where do you hurt? That's easy to answer; everyone knows where they hurt.

What were your sports in school? If he or she didn't go out for sports, you can usually assume a deficient musculature. Otherwise, you need only check the sports table in this book (Appendix 4) to find the muscles most likely to suffer.

Have you had or been in any accidents? Many people don't remember their accidents, and only later, when you find a really bad trigger point in an arm, say, you may hear, "Ouch, I just remembered I broke that arm in grade school."

Have you had any operations? Those they usually remember; the scars annoy them.

Have you any children? (Women get this one.) *How were they born?* If they had children, there will be trigger points in the pelvic area. If the children were forceps delivered, we ask about headaches. A frightening number of those children do have headaches.

What medications are you on? After you get this information check in the drug section

What were your occupations? See the table of occupations in Appendix 3 to see which muscles will have been "insulted."

Once the woman with chronic abdominal pain had filled out the question sheet for me I knew she'd been athletic, rode a lot, had never "worked," had had two children, had never been operated on, and had had the usual number of falls from horses. She did have a whiplash once, but it went away. With that information you don't have enough to go on until you ask one more question.

When was the first time you had the pain and what happened?

She'd had the pain for 35 years, and yes, she certainly remembered when it had started. She had had a hydrocephalic baby—one with an abnormal accumulation of fluid inside his skull which caused the skull to grow to an abnormal size and the brain to deteriorate. There was no hope for the baby, and they removed it piece by piece. This had been both painful and heartbreaking, and there had been abdominal pain ever since.

23

Now, with that information, you ask *yourself* the obvious questions.

Which muscles would be involved in such an event? The answer in this case was the abdominals, at least for a start.

Where do those muscles attach? They attach to the pubic arch at one end and to the ribs at the other.

With that information, I reached in under the rib cage and found a very tender spot just to the left of the sternum, or breastbone. You can see what I did on page 105. I held the pressure for the required seven seconds. When I took my hand away, she stretched the area by taking several deep breaths and then arching her back. She felt much better but was not completely painfree. Another trigger point was found on the opposite side. The stretches were done again with the help of a coolant spray. The pain was gone. Cheers! Wait up. Not quite—for I remembered that I had checked only one attachment, the sail end attached to the mast. What about the end attached to the boat? They were down in the pubic area. Trigger point pressure was applied, stretching exercises given, and a regular program of exercise provided, and the pain never came back.

What would have happened if we had overlooked the trigger points at the other end of the offending abdominals? An ignored matrix (and across the pubic arch they all feel like matrix points) would have been left there throbbing, and pretty soon some satellites would have carried the message back up to the trigger points I did get and the pain would have returned. Then Dr. Tivy, or whatever doctor had referred the patient for myotherapy, would probably have said, "Too bad, it doesn't work for that kind of pain . . ." But it does. If it is done right, it works for almost all chronic pain. And when it doesn't, the doctor should search further—for pathology.

MYOTHERAPY SUCCESS SCORE WITH CHRONIC PAIN: TO DATE, 95 PERCENT

Today some doctors are beginning to use myotherapy as a test, and that use has been pioneered by Dr. Tivy. If the patient with chronic back pain gets rid of it in one or two sessions, there isn't much sense in putting him or her through expensive tests. At the very least, the pain of the myelogram, in which a dye is injected into the spine, and the thumping headache that results, have been avoided.

X-rays aren't free either, nor are they free of peril. We are hearing more and more about the cumulative effects of radiation. Who knows, one day you may need a whole bunch. It's safer not to have used up your quota on X-rays that might have been avoided.

If myotherapy doesn't work, then the next step—tests—can be taken. But the success score to date for myotherapy at our institute is 95 percent.

4. Rid Yourself of Backache

Happily, the most common pain of all—backache—is the easiest to erase with myotherapy. The pain may be mild, like the slight discomfort experienced after a long drive, or it can be agonizing. Intractable back pain has driven people to suicide. When it strikes suddenly it can drop the sufferer senseless.

News Item: Seven million adults each lose ten to fifteen working days a year because of back pain.

ODYSSEY OF A BACKACHE SUFFERER

Let's consider that maddening backache that attacks suddenly and for no apparent reason. What to do?

If you are like most people, you gimp about for a week suffering, trying not to complain while eating aspirin and lying on an electric heating pad. You wait impatiently for the pain to go away, but it doesn't go so you go—to the doctor. You are given a prescription for a "muscle relaxant," plus a stronger analgesic than aspirin, and told to go to bed for at least 24 hours, "but a week would be smarter if you want to get better." You do go to bed and you don't feel any better. What next?

After the week in bed the pain is, if anything, a little worse so you are sent for X-ray. The X-rays are negative but you are still bent in half and groaning. The next step will be to the orthopedist. More X-rays will be ordered because very few doctors like other doctors' X-rays. Those, too, are negative and you don't know whether to be glad or sad. You decide on sad when your frustrated doctor sends you for more tests. The neurologist you see next has some good ones, all of which turn up negative, but now in addition to the backache you have a banging headache from the myelogram, the test involving injection of dye into the spine.

Since everything was negative, including the attitudes of the doctors who couldn't find a thing wrong with you, you are sent back to doctor number one who is now a triple failure. The first one couldn't help you, the selected orthopedist couldn't help you, the selected neurologist couldn't help you. What is the matter with you? The doctor's perplexity is as genuine as is the desire to help you. So, too, is the overriding wish to be rid of you so that the time can be given over to a couple of honest-to-God ulcer cases that *can* be helped.

Now, since there is obviously nothing wrong with your back (the tests all say so), it's probably up in your head along with the headache from the myelogram. Perhaps it will help to tranquilize you so that whatever is in your head will stop bothering you. You are given a fairly strong one, which you take along with the painkiller and the muscle relaxant (really another tranquilizer).

Still in pain but reluctant to go back to the first, second, or third doctor, you settle on a chiropractor. You feel better while he or she is doing whatever chiropractors do, but in a few days or even hours, there it is again, your old backache.

You begin to suspect cancer, a rare bone disease, disintegration of something or other. You wonder if they put the wrong X-rays in your envelope. You begin to think that *they* know, but are not telling you. Your stomach is upset. Is it spreading? Panic sets in, so you consult another doctor in another town. More X-rays. More tests. More referrals, until you are diagnosed as having "arthritis of the spine."

Now the very word *arthritis* has a stress effect and that's because arthritis equates with age and there's one thing you must not do in this society and that's age. Even death is preferable to aging. In your mind you see your end—hobbling along with a cane, back bent and feet shuffling, hairless, toothless, and, most probably, mindless.

The only good thing is that now at long last you have a name for your pain. And if there's a name, surely there's a cure? There is, but even if arthritis were the cause, you wouldn't care for the treatment, nor is it likely to get rid of the pain.

27

You would probably start with masses of aspirin tablets or something like Indocin, prednisone, or gold salts. They are very potent so you are not to be surprised if you feel under the weather for a few days. A few days! Feeling under the weather becomes a way of life, and pretty soon you notice that your skin has begun to wither and your hair to fall out. Since your depression deepens you get Ritalin to cheer you up. But now you can't sleep. No problem. Seconal was invented for just such a nuisance. By this time something will have happened for which there is no drug. Your sex life is nil, zilch, zero—gone. In time so is your husband, wife, or whatever. But you keep your wrinkled skin, your insomnia, and, especially, your backache.

And would you believe it was not arthritis that caused your pain in the first place? "Ah!" you say, "but it was. I saw it on the X-ray." Of course you saw it. It was there! If you look at X-rays of most people over 40 you will find some arthritis, but that's not what caused the pain, at least not directly and probably not at all.

There's another place to go if you develop chronic pain in your back, and that's to a psychiatrist's couch. That's not the worst place to be if you have an emotional upheaval, and most people with chronic pain lead stressful lives, but it won't cure the backache and it is awfully expensive.

There is still another way to try. After the psychiatrist fails to rid you of your pain (you are stubbornly attached to your neuroses), and the chiropractor, neurologist, orthopedist, and family doctor can do nothing more, you can go to a pain clinic.

Pain clinics are usually hospital connected and priced out of reality. Your stay will be a minimum of three weeks, and, if you can afford it, it may take months.

First you will be evaluated. All your X-rays will be examined, and, should you need more, you are in the right place. All the results of all your tests will be "evaluated" and ditto if you need additional ones.

Next you will be exposed to biofeedback, meditation, progressive relaxation, and behavior modification (because no doubt you want to keep your pain so you can enjoy the secondary payoffs like not having to go to work and like being the center of attention at the clinic).

The atmosphere where everyone is hurting and no one is making much progress becomes totally depressing. After a while you may feel low enough to settle on an exploratory operation even though most surgeons agree that an operation to locate pain is a wild goose chase. Worse, if it looks like you have a "slipped" disc, which really means ruptured, disintegrating, or degenerating disc, it will be removed.

With all the bother, cost, and discomfort of an operation, surely *now* the pain will go away. But it doesn't. You arise from your bed of pain still hurting.

And most of this suffering is unnecessary, because 95 percent of chronic back pain can be relieved.

Sometimes a disc really is at the root of the trouble, but all too often the patient is dismayed to find that after the operation is over and pronounced successful he or she is still plagued with pain.

A disc is the fibrocartilage acting as a cushion between the vertebrae. It is about 80 percent water, but as we get older the water content falls to about 70 percent and the disc loses some of its compressibility. This situation can set the stage for what is called a ruptured, or herniated, disc. In rare cases, such a rupture may bulge through the rear part of the outer ring and exert pressure on the nerves causing severe pain in the back, referring itself even all the way to the toes.

However, and this is a big *however*, at the Institute of Rehabilitation, New York University, Bellevue Medical Center, the doctors say that so many bad discs have been found in post mortems done on persons who never complained of back pain that the damaged disc can hardly be called the main villain.

One specialist, Dr. Paul Magnuson of Washington, D.C., a man with an enviable reputation, said some time ago, "I've only seen one ruptured disc out of every thousand so diagnosed in over forty years of working on backs. It's a meaningless term and obscures the cause and cure. Once upon a time everyone had 'sacroiliac trouble,' before that it was 'lumbago,' now it's 'discs.' "

No, the real villain isn't discs but a combination of these conditions: (1) chronic muscle deficiency from lack of exercise, (2) chronic strain due to poor musculature, and (3) chronic pain due to trigger points causing the inadequate muscles to go into spasms.

Chronic muscle deficiency is curable with exercise. Chronic muscle strain is preventable by building a better body. Ninety-five percent of chronic pain is reversible with myotherapy, exercise, good nutrition, and real physical education.

29

Back pain is often blamed on poor lifting habits. If so, how do you explain the fact that millions of Europeans do a lot of lifting, many have never heard of a "bent knee lift," but do not suffer with back pain, for instance, 90 percent of the Austrians?

Then there was the crime of leaning down with legs straight to pick up something from the floor. Quite a few agreed that was bad. But many people in Scandinavia milk their goats while leaning forward and down with legs straight not even bothering to squat on a milking stool. And they seldom have back pain.

Then there was the premise that women have more backaches than men because the curve in the female lumbar spine is more pronounced. Why then don't more Austrian women have backaches? They are just as female as women in the United States—sometimes even more so!

Americans are told not to overexert themselves because it can cause back pain. However, the Austrians, and other Europeans we have tested, the Swiss and Italians, for example, have to exert themselves in no small measure, yet their backache rate is far lower than ours. I do agree with the qualifying prefix *over*, that is, that no one should really overexert himself if it can be helped, but if we start out as children with a fitness level far below that needed for simple, daily living, almost everything will qualify as overexertion.

What can we do about back pain? Plenty!

Remember I said that a way has been found to erase most muscular pain. Please read on.

Here are step-by-step instructions, with accompanying illustrations, for finding and erasing the trigger points associated with the various back pains. Here too are directions for appropriate stretching exercises to help keep the back pains from acting up again.

We start by erasing the all-too-common, and maddening, lower back pain.

HOW TO ERASE LOWER BACK PAIN

We tell the youngsters who come to the institute that the trigger points for lower back pain are in the back pockets of their blue jeans. And that's where they are for your subject too—usually three or four to a "pocket."

To begin, have your subject strip down to underpants—preferably white briefs. Have him or her lie on the table face down. Now you are ready to tackle the first muscles, numbered 1, 2, and 3 on Plate 5 in Appendix 1. These muscles are in the buttocks (gluteals), more specifically, the gluteus maximus.

Reach across the body (this way you gain leverage), and place your elbow where the pocket would be. *Slowly* apply pressure. The pressure should *not* be straight down but angled back toward you, as shown in the picture.

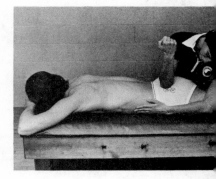

If your subject reacts (some try to fly right off the table), you have found a trigger point.

Hold the pressure on that spot for seven seconds.

After slowly withdrawing your elbow, you can (but it is not obligatory) mark x on the briefs at the exact spot from which you have just removed a trigger point. This will provide a useful record and will prevent you from pressing on the same area twice—for which your friend on the table will be most grateful. You can, of course, just mark your map.

If there is no reaction to your elbow's pressure, the trigger point is not where your elbow is. So, without changing the degree of pressure, move your elbow around a bit. Somewhere near there you will hit pay dirt. Mark your x on briefs and/or your map.

Try for two more trigger points in the same "pocket" area and record x's in the same way.

Lori demonstrates a useful technique. She weighs one hundred pounds wringing wet and Rick, her subject, is six feet two. In order for her to probe deep enough into his muscles she uses her left arm to help generate extra pressure. By clasping her hands together she can use the power of both arms on one elbow.

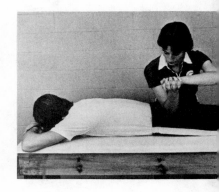

To get an idea of how your probing feels to the subject, close your eyes and press the sharp end of a pencil into your thigh. You are well aware of where the point is and how hard you are pressing. You may even wonder whether it will break the skin. A sharp elbow planted on one's gluteals, where there are sure to be very tender spots, feels about the same. And when the elbow hits a trigger point, it will feel as though it has a nail sticking out from the end.

Now close your eyes and press the pencil into your thigh, but surround the point with your other hand which you lay flat against your thigh. Press both at the same time and the pain will

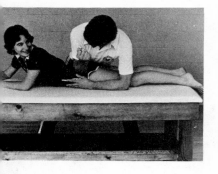

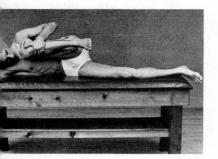

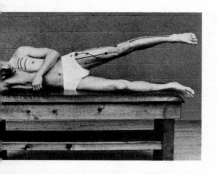

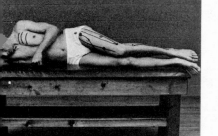

be diffused. Lori, who is little, covers some of the trigger point area with her own body, as you can see in the photograph on page 36.

Rick, who is both big and strong enough to find any trigger point with one elbow, surrounds the entire area with his body and one arm, thus softening the pain.

When you have found and defused the trigger points in the gluteus maximus, remember that at least part of the spasm has been released. Now the muscle lies there, not sure what to do. It's been in a shortened, tense position so long it is unable to let go, so you have to help it. You must show it how to relax, and you do that by stretching it.

SIDE-LYING STRETCH EXERCISE
Have your friend roll over onto one side, *slowly*. The muscle you have just cleared is so confused that a sudden movement might cause it to jump back into the same mess from which you just rescued it.

You may or may not have to help with the exercise, but it is just as well to assist the first three or four times to make sure your friend knows exactly what you want.

This exercise stretches the gluteals you have just cleared. It also stretches the muscles all down the back. Do these exercises slowly and with a rhythm. Muscles "listen" to rhythm. In the photographs for this exercise and other exercises, you can see that Rick has been marked up to help you locate muscles and trigger points. There is no need to mark your subject, however.

1. Draw the top knee up to the chest.
2. Extend the leg straight down about eight inches above the resting leg.
3. Rest the raised leg on the resting leg. Relax for a slow count of three.

If your subject is a gymnast or a dancer, he or she will tend to point the toes. This is not good because it tightens the leg muscles. Be sure the subject's toes are not pointed. Do the exercise four times.

Remember, the body has two sides. Since you found trigger points on one side, there are probably some on the other, even though only one side hurts. Cross over to your subject's other side and do the other "pocket." Then repeat the exercise with the other leg.

ERASING TRIGGER POINTS FROM HIPS

The muscle we tackle here, the gluteus medius, is on either side of the pelvis. (See spots 4, 5, and 6 on Plate 6 in Appendix 1.) If your subject were wearing warm-up pants, it would be right under the top part of the stripe running down each leg.

Incidentally, there's a bonus to be had from erasing trigger points from this muscle. If followed with fibrositis massage (see under Fibrositis Massage in Chapter 7) plus some of the hip exercises (see under Your Basic Fitness Program to Keep Pain Away in Chapter 10), it will help reduce that unsightly hip line called "saddle bags."

The pressure required for this muscle must be applied straight down, not at an angle to the body. To do it right is a bit tricky and will need good control. Be careful not to let your elbow slide off to either side.

It is not important whether you start with spot 4, 5, or 6 on the chart. And since there is less flesh between your elbow and the subject's pelvis, less pressure will be required than in the thicker buttocks muscle.

Have the subject lie on his or her side with the knees slightly bent. Search out trigger points. There are usually three between the waist and the bottom line of the subject's briefs. These trigger points often come under the heading of "awful."

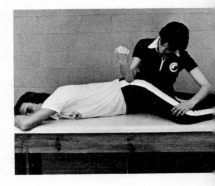

Hold the pressure in each spot for the usual seven seconds. Mark your x's as you find and erase the trigger points. Follow with this exercise.

CROSS-LEG STRETCH

While the subject remains in the same position, press the top leg forward and down to stretch the gluteus medius and the muscle along the outside of the thigh, namely the vastus lateralis (shown in Plate 9) which shares this exercise.

Place one of your hands on the crest of the subject's pelvis at the waist, and with the other, press down on the knee in eight short, easy bounces.

When you have cleared both sides of trigger points and done the cross-leg stretch on both sides, go back and repeat the side-lying stretch, described earlier in this chapter.

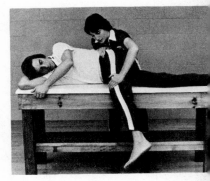

33

MUSCLES OF THE BACK AND BACK PAIN

Most people with back pain are sure the trouble is in the spine. The truth is that it rarely is. Of course, disc problems do exist, but many doctors are trying rest and exercise first and surgery only as a last resort. The trouble with rest is that it leads to something with a great name, post-inertial-dyskinesia. What all that means is that it's painful to start moving after you have been sitting or lying for a while. The pain that results is also called "jelling pain."

There are also conditions with names like scoliosis, kyphosis, and others, which describe a spine being pulled out of line. But, one might ask, what's doing the pulling? Bones can't go anywhere by themselves. It's muscles that make them work. We know that when muscles contract they pull. If the muscles on one side of the back are bigger and stronger than the corresponding muscles on the other side, something has to give. If the muscles on one side are shorter, that is, more contracted, than those on the other, something has to give. What gives is the spine, and we think trigger points are doing it.

Moreover, the muscles that can cause trouble in the back are so numerous that it really makes more sense to consider them first, not the 24 little vertebrae that catch all the hell and figure into too many diagnoses.

ERASING TRIGGER POINTS FROM THE "BELT" AREA

You have worked in the "pockets" of blue jeans and down the "stripes" of warm-up pants; now let's examine the back and sides of the "belt." Once again the technique changes a little.

Stand or sit with your hands at your waist, thumbs facing forward, fingers touching your spine and palms flat on your back. Arch your back slightly. As the back muscles contract, there will be two bulges of muscle, one in the palm of each hand. You are going to work on both sides of each of those bulges and each time toward the middle of the bulge. (In the following illustration, note the two bulges of muscle on either side of Rick's spine.)

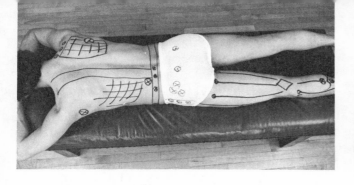
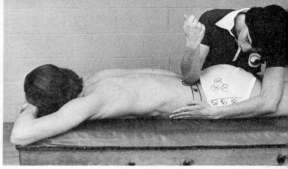

Have your subject lie on the table, face down. Think of your subject's belt as studded with four stars on each side. They are numbered 7, 8, 9, and 10 on Plate 5 in Appendix 1. The first star (that is, possible trigger point) you will examine is on the outside of one of those bulges about four inches from the spine, number 8, the second one out from the spine. Stand on the side *away* from the muscle to be searched. Reach across your subject's body and place your elbow against the far side of the muscle. Press down and pull toward you as if trying to get in under the bulge of the muscle.

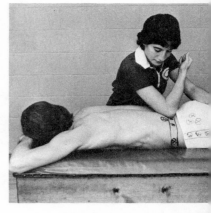

The second star to be worked is spot 7, next to the spine. Place your elbow against the bulge and push down and *outward*. Sometimes those muscles shield trigger points, especially in athletes, and you want to be sure you leave no fifth columnists to stir up trouble later.

Move your elbow about one inch outward past spot 8 on the same horizontal belt line and repeat what you did with the first star, this time on spot 9. Press down and pull toward you.

The last star, spot 10, on the muscle called the external oblique on the side away from you, requires a slightly different technique. For all the others the trigger points were found between a bone structure and your elbow or a thick mass and your elbow. This spot is just below the rib cage and just above the bony rim of the pelvis and is very vulnerable in any twisting action, which is required in most sports, for example, batting, the golf swing, and the twisting turn when catching a basketball. This area is often damaged if you are in a car skid, and it should always be checked even when your X-rays are negative. Reach across the back and about halfway down the side toward the table. Then pull toward you *and up*. This is the only upward motion you ever use with your elbow.

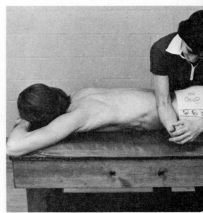

Erase any trigger points you find and mark your *x*'s.

When you have "cleared" one side of the belt area you will need to stretch the muscles with this exercise.

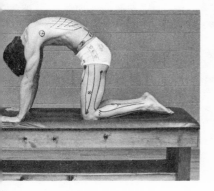

CAT BACK-OLD HORSE STRETCH EXERCISE

Have your subject get on hands and knees and press the back upward like an angry cat while dropping the head down. There is a tendency to bend the arms slightly. Don't let that happen.

Next, let the back fall in as though it belonged to a tired, old sway-backed horse. Bring the head up and be sure the arms are still straight.

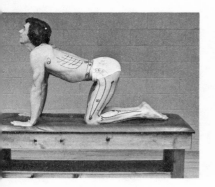

Do this exercise four times, always slowly and with great concentration, searching out all the tight spots that need to be stretched.

Now cross over to the other side of your subject, erase trigger points in the belt area on the opposite side, mark your x's, and repeat the stretch exercise. If you had the condition called "sciatica," in which there is pain radiating down either or both legs, in all probability it is gone. Sciatica is thought to be caused by a nerve being "pinched." A nerve is indeed being pinched, but in most cases not by the spine. The nerve has its little tail in a crack all right, but a muscle in spasm is doing the pinching. We have not had a single case of sciatica in five years that didn't get better when we did what you have just done.

The last island of trouble in the belt area is spot 11 (shown in Plate 5), which is above the belt between the second and third stars. Use the same type of pressure as that used for spot 9.

THE LIMBERING SERIES

This exercise program is a must for all ex-back sufferers. When your back is no longer a bother, add this complete series of back limbering exercises to your daily routine.

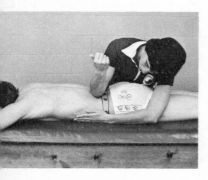

If you are on maintenance with this series (which means you no longer have pain), do one complete series morning and night.

If you still have some pain from time to time, try to get it in four times daily.

If you are still very close to the "bad days," try to do the series twice, three to four times a day, or even oftener if you can. It's your back.

1. *Supine Stretch*

Lie supine with knees bent and arms resting at your sides. Raise your head and bring the left knee as close to your nose as you can. You may (should) help the stretch with your hands. Lie back and stretch the left leg out straight about ten inches above the bed or floor. Return to the beginning position and relax for three seconds. Alternate legs, doing the exercise four times on each side.

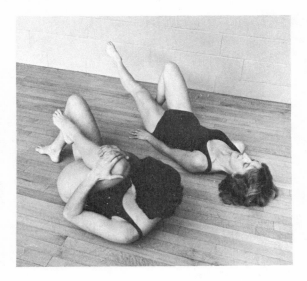

2. *Side-Lying Stretch*

Roll over onto your *right* side and take a comfortable, relaxed position. Draw the left knee up as close to your chest as you can. Stretch the leg down, parallel with the resting leg and about eight inches above it. Lower the leg and rest for three seconds. Repeat four times, on this side only. Doing it on the other side comes later in the routine.

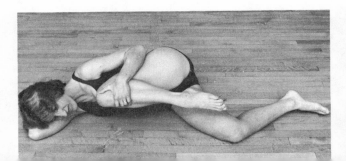 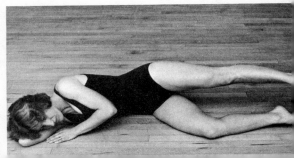

3. Prone Gluteal and Abdominal Set

Roll over until you are prone, with your head resting on your bent arms. Tighten your seat muscles (gluteals) and your abdominals. Hold for five seconds, then relax for three seconds. Repeat three more times.

At this point, continue to roll in the direction you started, stop when you are on your left side, and repeat the side-lying exercise on this side.

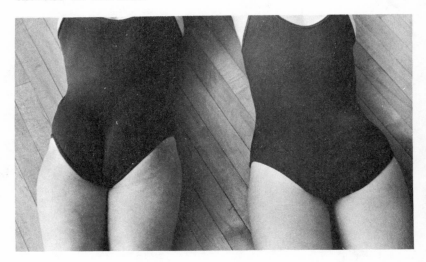

4. Supine Pelvic Tilt

Finish the roll onto your back with knees bent and feet about eighteen inches apart. Arch the back slightly keeping both seat and shoulders touching the floor. Then press the spine down hard while tilting the pelvis under as far as possible. Hold the tilt for five seconds and relax. Repeat four times.

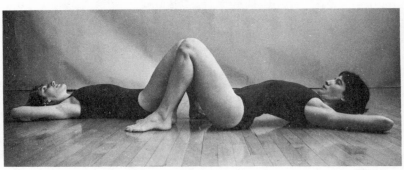

Rid Yourself of Headaches and Jaw Pain

5.

Most headaches are curable, and almost all the rest of them are controllable. Only about 5 percent of persistent head pain can be labeled pathological. Let's leave that 5 percent to the doctors. When all pathology has been ruled out but the headache remains, we can be almost sure it's myotherapy's baby.

When headaches are caused by trigger points (and we believe most of them are), the original cause can be any one of the many things we have talked about: your birth, an accident, your participation in sports, any of your several occupations. And who knows, maybe your stint as a free-lance typist 20 years ago contributed a few trigger points along with the cash for college.

Disease, even when under control, can cause headaches. Any fall involving the head can cause headaches, and that means almost any fall because the head is the tip of the whip that snaps.

Some headaches are laid at the door of heredity. If yours is just like the one suffered by dear old Dad, you may think it is inherited. Stop thinking that way. Dad could have given you his sky-blue eyes, but he didn't give you his headache.

Who has headaches? Dr. Howard Kurland, Professor of Psychiatry at Northwestern University, says that more than 90 percent of all American adults and teenagers are afflicted with headache at one time or other. Other experts hold that 90 percent suffer at least one headache every 30 days.

What kinds of headaches are these people said to have? They will tell you they have "sinus headaches," "tension headaches," "sick headaches," "eyestrain headaches," "constipation headaches," "allergy headaches," "menstrual headaches," "hangover headaches," "fever headaches," and even "weekend headaches." There is also the headache no one likes to mention, the "no-sex-tonight headache." Twelve million people in this country are said to be handicapped by what are referred to as migraine headaches. All headaches are bad, but migraines are usually worse.

Migraine has been known to medical science for at least two thousand years. The Roman physician Galen named it hemicrania ("half the head") because it attacks only one side of the face or skull. In the Middle Ages it was re-named "megrim," a term we now use for low spirits, blind staggers, and a general feeling of misery. Today we have the word migraine. By whatever name, however, migraines attack one side of the head.

What is a migraine like? It is said to be a blinding pain often accompanied by nausea, vomiting, visual disturbances, lack of coordination, dizziness, bloating of the stomach, fainting spells, and even numb or tingling hands. A shocking 2 percent of our population or about four million people have those headaches on a regular basis.

The two important categories of migraine are classic migraine and common migraine. The classic is different from the common only in the phase that precedes the attack. In a classic migraine the sufferer experiences prodromal symptoms. These can range from physical problems such as seeing auras or flashing lights, distorted hearing, and loss of coordination, to emotional imbalance. It is the prodromata or foreshadowing symptoms that scare sufferers sometimes to the point of madness. They hear things that can't be there, like the pounding of the sea, bells ringing, whips crackling, or bees buzzing. Sometimes vision is blurred or blind spots occur. Parts of the body can feel as though they are expanding while others seem to shrink. Some people feel as though they are leaving the body altogether and taking off on an astral trip.

SOME THEORIES ON THE CAUSES OF MIGRAINES

It is thought that migraines are vascular problems and are caused when arteries within the skull expand. Then the arteries "pull" on the nerves surrounding them. It is this pulling that is believed to cause the pain. Other experts feel that there is a decrease in the flow of blood to the brain, causing impairment of its function. One widely believed possibility is that substances within the brain called bradykinin and serotonin, which are known to cause pain, may suddenly accumulate. Still other people believe migraines are activated by a virus. We have a different idea. We think that migraine headaches, like most other headaches, are caused by trigger points. To understand how this could be, let's look at the head.

Most people haven't the slightest idea of how the head is made, or what besides the brain is in there. While there are only a limited number of pain-sensitive nerves inside the head, it is surrounded by many. The external covering consists of skin and scalp, both of which are well supplied with nerve endings and many, many blood vessels. A scalp wound can be superficial and yet bleed copiously, as any mother knows who has raced her screaming, bleeding offspring to the emergency room.

Beneath the scalp lie the bones of the skull that protect the brain, which floats in a sac of fluid called the cerebrospinal fluid. The sac and its fluid encase both the brain and the extension of the brain, the spinal cord, which goes down through the backbone all the way to its base.

While there are millions of nerve fibers in the head and brain, there are only twelve pairs of cranial nerves that come directly from the brain. They serve important areas of the head, the sense organs, and the upper chest cavity.

There are also motor nerves which feed instructions from the brain to the muscles and glands.

A third group consists of sensory nerves which receive impulses to the brain. One of the pairs is called trigeminal because it has three main branches. Each of the main branches has accessory branches that run throughout the face and head carrying both pain and temperature messages all over the head, the mucous membranes of the mouth, the teeth, and the meninges, which make up the sac protecting the brain. It is no wonder at all that the face and head are so sensitive, and it is easy to see how pain can be transferred from one part of the head to another.

Not long ago we had a man at a pain erasure clinic who was suffering from facial pains caused by trouble in the trigeminals. His face was all bruised from alcohol injections made in an

41

effort to block the nerve. They hadn't. The myotherapist tried on the first day to locate the offending trigger points and was unsuccessful. The next day a second myotherapist was working opposite a dentist who said, "You know, sometimes when I inadvertently press on a place *in* the mouth the patient says he feels better. . . . Do you think? . . ."

They both dashed for the washrooms to wash their hands. In the mouth, they found the trigger points that were affecting the teeth. Soon all that was left was pain in the lower lip. That responded to myotherapy as well. The pain was gone. You really don't know what myotherapy will do until you try it.

Migraine and Trigger Points

Trigger points are in muscles, right? When you look at your head, or better, a bald head, you don't see any muscles, do you? But wait! There really are lots of muscles in your head and face.

Suppose you break your cheekbone when in an accident you bang it against the dashboard. Take a minute to study Plates 12 through 15 in Appendix 1 showing the head bones and face muscles. Just imagine what that simple fracture (you may not even know you broke something) involves in the way of potential trigger points, from the chest, along the neck, over the entire head, and down into the shoulders.

Headaches and Pressure on Blood Vessels

It is believed that the greatest source of head pain stems from the blood vessels that lead to and from the brain. It is true that the brain uses 25 percent of the body's entire blood supply at any one time, so there is a strong basis for that belief. It is further believed that the blood vessels cause so much trouble because they are so richly supplied with pain-sensitive nerves. And finally it is thought that most headaches are directly related to changes in pressure or size of the blood vessels.

If pain is caused by pressure on the blood vessels, what is causing the pressure? I have a theory and it's as good as anyone else's until proved wrong. I think muscles in spasm put the blood vessels under pressure. We have known for a long time that when legs are freed of spasms, varicose veins subside and feet get warm. Spasm, it would seem, puts pressure on the blood vessels and denies the legs and feet an adequate oxygen supply. On the other hand, when muscles are free of spasm and the vessels free of pressure, there is a good supply of blood to the extremities. Feet will be warm and free from pain, and it doesn't matter if the subject is in a king-size bed or a narrow ledge on the Matterhorn. There will be no leg cramps.

In the same way, I believe, pressure on blood vessels in and around the head can cause headaches. In your head, nerves travel every which way while muscles are strapped over, under, and around other muscles. Think of how vulnerable the head is, how much abuse it has taken from birth on, and all the trigger points that have been accumulated. Think of how frequently triggering mechanisms occur, from bumping another kid's head to getting a bridge that doesn't quite fit. Perhaps you grind your teeth at night, or are addicted to chewing gum, a pipe, or your own nails. Think of how often you are under stress, even pleasurable stress. My father-in-law was delighted with the forthcoming marriage of his oldest son, but just as the guests walked in the door he got the wildest migraine imaginable.

There are thought to be five commonly recognized types of migraines, or vascular headaches. All of them strike me as having a similar cause, that is, trigger points, which force muscles into spasm, which in turn prevents the free flow of blood to the head and can also press on nerves.

We have discussed classic and common migraines. The following type is said to be so painful that it has been known to lead to suicide.

Cluster Headache

This is thought to come on as the result of a sudden production of histamine, a chemical produced by the body. The headaches have a peculiar "clustering" characteristic—a sharp pain in the temple or behind the eye. This is followed by a painfree period, only to be followed by more pain. We feel that histamine may well activate trigger points the same way alcohol does.

Hemiplegic and Ophthalmoplegic Migraine

Hemiplegia means weakness or paralysis of one side, and ophthalmoplegia means paralysis or weakness of the eye muscles, resulting in double vision.

43

Henry was a tall Texan who drove a moving van for a living. He was huge, dark skinned, with dark eyes and was the very picture of what Pancho Villa should have looked like. He was also in agony and had been for nearly 20 years. During the last three years the level of pain had been mounting, and finally he could bear no more.

Twenty years before he came to the institute, Henry had been hit by a car. His back, left hip, and left leg were severely damaged as were his head, neck, left arm, and left shoulder. His eyesight was affected and occasionally he had double vision— just what you need when driving a loaded moving van down highway I-95 on a rainy night.

One day he heard me talking to Arlene Francis on the radio about the relief of pain. Right away he set about getting a load to be moved to Massachusetts. He and his wife arrived, and the work began. The first day he felt "a little better." Next morning, when asked the most important question that can follow a session, "How did you sleep?" he answered, "Fine. Fine, for the first time in many years." Relaxation during sleep speaks volumes. It is definitive evidence of a significant change.

The second day he was "much better" when he left. While most painful backs and legs, even heads, necks, and arms, surrender after two sessions, a shoulder takes longer. Also, the pain had been at full force for 20 years. "Could he possibly stay over for one more day?" we asked. They decided to stay.

That evening some of the staff were having dinner at a Berkshire inn, when in they walked. No one could miss them. He, looking all of his six feet four, was dressed in western clothes all in white and covered with turquoise and silver. She, too, glowed with silver and turquoise. They spotted us, and there was no stopping him. He rushed over and stood at the table trying to say something, but unable to find the words. Instead he started to cry, no sound, just huge tears rolling down. Finally he found the words, "I don't hurt anywhere. Anywhere."

Later, on leaving, we stopped by their table. "Look at him!" said his wife. "Just look at him. He hasn't had to get up from the table *once*!" When one suffers from back and/or hip pain, it is often impossible to sit through a meal without getting up to relieve the spasm. Henry hadn't sat through a meal for 20 years.

The next day when Henry's third session was over and while his myotherapist was giving his wife some final instructions on what to do if he hurt, he suddenly leaned over and picked up one of the publications from the table. He looked as though he had just read something startling. It was startling all right. *He could see to read.* That joy also had been missing for 20 years.

Please understand: If there are sight changes due to disease, removing any trigger points that may be present will not make any difference in your vision. However, if sight problems are caused by a lack of proper circulation, it can. We have correspondence with a blind woman in Utah whose doctor told her that her problem was circulatory. Her best treatment would be walking five miles a day. But how, pray tell, is a solitary woman, blind and living alone, going to manage five miles a day on the roads of Utah?

We wrote back sending a map of the trigger points to be hunted down and extinguished. Within three weeks she wrote back, "I can now see to dial a phone number. . . ."

If the cause of blindness is imperfect circulation due to muscle spasm, the first move is to get rid of the spasm, but that must be followed by exercise. The five-mile walk is often impractical, but I have put together a four-hour program on records for use by people with impaired vision. It is called *Physical Fitness for You.* (See the Sources section for details on ordering.) It is without question the best exercise record I have done and can be used by anyone, even those confined to a wheelchair. One need not be completely blind to use it either, just visually impaired, and wanting a better life.

Down Migraine

Down migraine is not a separate type of migraine. Its name refers to when it occurs. It is said to attack after a period of stress. This headache is sometimes likened to the depression that sets in after a mountainous "high." A down headache is likely to arrive promptly on Saturday morning after a pistol of a week. My feeling about this one is that there are trigger points in residence. The sufferer has a built-in time table (we all do). He or she must squash fatigue, temperament, and that *Oh-my-god-I'll-never-make-it* feeling, then go ahead and make it anyway. After the job is done, something inside says, "OK, so collapse." People who don't have trigger points in their head muscles, faces, and necks can go to bed and sleep 14 hours. Those who do end up with down migraine instead.

45

OTHER KINDS OF HEADACHE

Nervous Headache

Leaving "vascular" headaches behind, we come to the muscle-contraction headache, also called a nervous headache. Either name you call this beauty mentions a part of the trium-virate causing pain: muscle spasm—contraction caused by trigger points, "nerves" resulting from a stressful climate, with the third part, the triggering mechanism, free for the choosing. There is never enough aspirin in a college town at exam time. An unpleasant visit with an unpleasant relative can set up a nifty. One more spilled glass of milk will do it, as will one more slammed door.

Sinus Headache and Trigger Points

When my children were small it was fashionable to have sinus headache, or sinus drip. People carried nose drops or little nasal squirt guns, and according to prescription, every hour or two dropped or squirted. Today this condition is usually called an allergy or a reaction to stress. I agree.

There are two things to be done to clear up the condition. First, clear the sinuses (see under Erasing Trigger Points Around the Nose and Cheekbones, later in this chapter), and second, look to the emotional climate. Remember, you may have made that bed but you don't have to lie in it forever. If there is someone in it you can't stand, take action!

Hangovers and Other Normally Nonrecurring Headaches

This type, nonmigrainous vascular, is said to result from swelling or dilation of the arteries within the skull from causes which do not usually recur. Carbon monoxide poisoning, food poisoning, hangovers, coffee-withdrawal reactions, and high blood pressure are examples.

I would hope that carbon monoxide poisoning would not be a recurrent cause. Symptoms from coffee withdrawal at least can be linked to their cause since no real coffee drinker can give it up without knowing it. Coffee-withdrawal headache may well be a triggering mechanism rather than a cause for pain. I would look for trigger points. High blood pressure might be the cause of head pain. It would be worth a trip to the doctor to have the pressure checked. If it is too high, medication is available, but diet and exercise are too, and they have no side effects.

As for hangovers, we have had considerable response from the college crowd when a pain erasure session was advertised simply like this:

```
HELP YOUR FRIENDS . . .
LEARN TO CURE HANGOVERS
```

An anti-hangover session usually lasts 15 minutes, with the cure effected by extinguishing trigger points in the head, face, and neck that were fired by alcohol.

"Referred" Headaches

Then there is a group of headaches said to be referred from various other head areas—eye, ear, nose, sinus, or dental structures. This group deserves serious attention.

You already know that matrix trigger points can affect, or in myotherapy parlance, "refer to," other parts of the body quite a distance from their own abodes. There is no question but that trouble in the neck muscles can refer to the head. They can easily cause eye, ear, tooth, and jaw pain, even dizziness. Trigger points around the eyes can cause head pain and vice versa. Just how often this happens is described later in this chapter when we discuss TMJD—temporomandibular joint dysfunction.

CHECK FOR ABNORMALITIES

At this point, it should be reiterated that acute pain is a warning. Pain tells you to check with the doctor. There are such things as brain tumors. True, there is less than one percent occurrence of brain tumor among headache sufferers, but if it is there, it can be, and must be, found and dealt with. Abnormal conditions within the skull can be located with CAT scans (computerized axial tomography). There are also X-rays to locate fractures and the EEG (electroencephalogram) to check for abnormal brain waves. If the source of pain remains elusive, there is still the angiogram, in which a dye is injected before X-ray. There are also lumbar punctures, spinal taps, and tests using radio-

47

isotopes. There are any number of tests that will find the trouble, if indeed trouble there is.

Be sure to have your doctor check for the possible causes for head pain: hypoglycemia, diabetes, kidney disease, hypertension, a fall, or a blow to the head. There are nondestructive ways to check them all out. There are many tools that in the hands of experts will uncover the cause for pathology, and as mentioned earlier, about 5 percent of head pains are caused by serious conditions.

MYOTHERAPY RECORD: 95 PERCENT SUCCESS

Ninety-five percent of the time, however, if you think your headache comes from trigger points, triggering mechanism, and climate, you will be right on target. Whatever the name given the pain—vascular, tension, sinus, nervous—it's still just a headache. Try a "head hunt" and examine the climate. Maybe you really should go to school, leave school, get a job, write a book, get married, get unmarried, fire the cook, hire a maid, join a group, resign from a group, go to India or Ceylon—or Brooklyn. Only you can decide whether or not your bed is not only bearable, but comfortable.

Now that we have discussed the kinds of headaches—all miserable—it's time to learn about a few people who have had them.

Craig was fifteen and had had "migraines" since he was six. He spent roughly one week out of four in bed, saw stars, and threw up all over school and home the day the headaches came on. Craig missed his sophomore year in high school because of his headaches. He had had every test and tried every medication, and nothing helped. No medication did more than reduce the pounding throbs to a dull ache. And when he was on the drug, he was off everything else, including school. "Did he ever have a fall?" His mother said no, not that she remembered. "But he did bump heads with another little boy when he was four and had a terrible lump on his forehead. Funny thing," she said, "his forehead still swells when he gets a headache." That was the clue. Trigger points, very active in the site of the original "insult." It took one hour to rid Craig of his headache. His mother was taught the technique and worked with him at home. Craig came back to us, once a month, twice more. He no longer has "migraines." He is able to participate in sports in school, denied him before, and has even become a proficient skier.

Nancy is a waitress. That fact says volumes. The physical strain of carrying trays, the stress of dealing with the public, and the triggering mechanism of moving fast on varying surfaces are omnipresent.

Nancy had had migraines for seventeen years. Every working day of the year she went to a chiropractor after she was through at the job. She was also through for the evening, laid up with a throbbing headache on the right side of her head. Medication was a way of life. After all, you can't wait on tables with your face in a knot and your last meal in danger of ejection. Dr. Tivy sent her over.

With Nancy it was even easier than with Craig. It was harder however to *keep* her painfree, because like the little girl who fell off her horse with predictable regularity, Nancy's work took its toll daily. Another on-the-site maintenance crew was required. This time a daughter became the crew. Missy, then eleven, now thirteen, was given instruction. The headaches are gone and Missy has become very skillful. At the first sign of a throb or squint, her little hands go to work, nor does she confine her efforts to Nancy. There are three brothers and sisters and innumerable friends who are painfree because a little girl's mother had headaches.

Timmy was six. He had come to a workshop with his mother, and after the children's class, which is notable for all its running, jumping, tumbling, and general excitement, I was talking about erasing headaches. "You mean," said Timmy's mother, "you can take headaches away just like that?" I said, "Yes, usually." "Well here's a little boy crying with a headache. He always gets them when he plays hard. Can you help him?" With Timmy it took only ten minutes, probably because it was a young headache. "How fast was he born?" I asked. "Oh, very fast. None of my younger ones came fast." Fast birth usually means very hard contractions. Hard contractions subject little heads to hard knocks. Hard knocks "insult" head muscles, and trigger points are born along with the baby.

And lastly—Dr. Tivy wanted to have us demonstrate the technique for the director of a noted Headache Research Center, so he invited him to come and watch. We had never seen the two patients who had been asked to take part in the demonstration, but both had long histories of head pain. One was a girl of ten who had been hit in the head with a baseball bat two years before. The question of cause was clear. The second case was not so clear unless one is trained to listen, and to ask the right questions. Background: Tomboy (that translates to falls, bumps, bruises, and a competitive nature); horsewoman (remember the little girl?); bookkeeper (that means tension and close work); plus the added daily strain of heaving hundred-pound bales of hay around a horse barn.

Under the watchful eyes of the doctors we erased these two chronic headaches in 40 minutes. The little girl has been fine ever since. Didi, the bookkeeper, was back with one of the worst headaches of her life the following week. Nausea, auras, and agonizing pain. She was desperate; we were not. Often taking away the armoring spasm we mentioned earlier uncovers deeper layers of trouble which then must be erased. In one hour one of the newest apprentices at the institute had changed the gray-faced, squinting woman into a different person. She came down the hall with the nurse who had brought her from work. Her eyes were wide and sparkling, her face rosy and relaxed. Pain gone, she was changed. Everyone is a different person when painfree. Six months, twenty-four payrolls (Didi always got a headache when making up a payroll), and six menstrual periods (another headache triggering mechanism) have passed with not a single throb—and Didi had what was called classic migraine.

"HEAD-HUNTING" IN SEARCH OF PAIN

So what do we do? We start with the premise that a headache by any name is still a headache and that, except for that other 5 percent, a headache can be erased at best and controlled at worst. Controlled means that headaches return from time to time, but before they get into full swing they can be aborted with myotherapy.

We treat all headaches the same way and most of the time begin with orbicularis oculi. Look at Plate 12 in Appendix 1 and you will see that skinless, we all look like owls, with those round eyes. The muscle circling the eye, the orbicularis, harbors many trigger points.

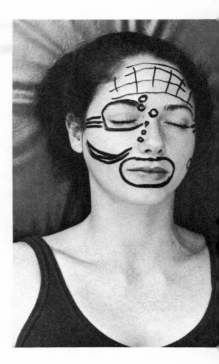

ERASING TRIGGER POINTS AROUND THE EYES

The lines on Chris's face represent the lines you will work along, searching for trigger points. The large circles around the eye and mouth are to be followed as you work around given areas. The small circles represent specific trigger point areas. Trigger points in the muscles in those spots produce facial changes and expressions, none of them good. The grids mark areas every point of which must be checked out.

What we need first is the technique. The tools for the face, neck, and head come with the operator; they are his or her fingers, knuckles, and thumbs. The knuckles are used in two ways: first, to press against a known trigger point, and second, in what is called the roller technique. The latter is a better way to cover a large area, such as a grid, than by poking with a finger in every last square inch. A fist is made, and you roll the knuckles over the area starting with the knuckle of the index finger and ending with the knuckle of the little finger. If you encounter no sensitive spots, good! No trigger points. If you do, stop right then and hold the pressure for five seconds. The roller technique is illustrated in the photograph on page 54.

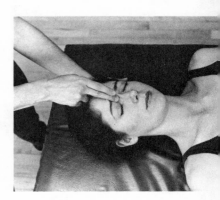

The wraparound technique employs the index finger on the face, the entire hand on the ribs, or both hands on the pelvis. The finger, hand, or hands press the muscle against bone by wrapping it over the bone edge. In the photograph on the next page you can see that the eyebrow is being pushed down over the socket edge, but check the illustration in the section on menstrual cramps, page 105, and you can see it better.

Have the subject lie on his or her back with eyes closed while you stand at the end of the table behind the subject's head. Using your index finger press upward against the edge of the bony socket. You are working on spot 61 as shown on Plate

12 in Appendix 1. Use about 6 pounds pressure and hold for five seconds. Then circle around the eye on that line pressing at finger-width intervals.

You have been working on the orbicularis oculi, which closes the eyelids, wrinkles the forehead, and compresses the lacrimal sac.

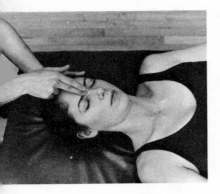

When you have completed circling both eyes, have the subject close the lids and, keeping the eyes closed, raise the eyebrows as high as possible, then scrunch up the entire face. Relax and repeat three more times.

Next we search for trigger points on the outer edge of the same muscle, spot 61 on Plate 12 in Appendix 1. Here we use the wraparound technique. Again use the index finger, or the middle finger if it is stronger.

Place your finger at the *top edge* of the eyebrow and, pressing gently, push the muscle downward until it wraps around the rim of the eye socket. Circle both eyes as before, pressing at finger-width intervals.

Repeat the above exercise and add one more.

With the eyes still closed have the subject look left, right, up, and down. Rest and repeat.

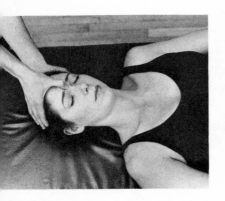

When you used the wraparound technique on the upper side of the orbicularis oculi, you included the corrugator. This muscle draws the eyebrow downward and medially. When you pressed at the inside corner of the eye you included the depressor supercilii, the one that depresses the eyebrow. Since pain causes wincing and frowning, you can see why an overworked wince or frown can contribute even more trigger points to cause even more pain.

We go on now to clear the trigger point at spot 62, shown on Plate 12. Place your thumb directly between the eyes, just above the bridge of the nose. Press firmly. Hold for five seconds. This muscle, the procerus, also draws the eyebrow down, which is one reason for raising the eyebrow as a stretch exercise.

ERASING TRIGGER POINTS AROUND THE NOSE AND CHEEKBONES

Along the sides of the nose there are two opposing muscles, the nasalis and the levator labii superioris alequae nasi. When the former contracts, it pulls the nasal wing downward and backward and reduces the size of the nostril. It produces a happy, astonished expression. We don't use it enough. The latter elevates the nasal wing and enlarges the nostrils. The facial expression thus produced is one of displeasure and discontent. Every time you show anger, or disgust, that muscle cramps tight. If the muscle houses a trigger point your anger could trigger a headache. So what do we do about it?

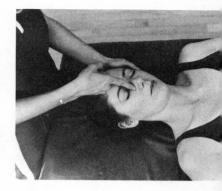

We start at spot 63, as shown on Plate 12, and press against the side of the nose at adjacent spots from top to bottom, holding for five seconds at each spot where a trigger point is encountered. Your finger will be wide enough to cover both muscles.

To stretch those muscles, pull them laterally toward the cheeks with two fingers on each side.

You will find that these muscles, when freed of trigger points, will present you with a bonus: Very often your stuffy nose will start to run and pressure will seem to clear away from the sinus areas.

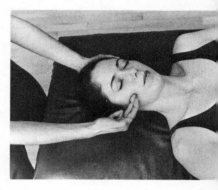

The cheek bone serves as a good marker for line A (see Plate 12). As we press at finger width *upward* against the cheek bone we trap the zygomaticus major muscle, which draws the mouth backward and upward. That could be part of a facial expression of laughter and pleasure, but then, it could also be one of pain, even agony. Under your fingers will also be the zygomaticus minor, the muscle that draws the lip upward and laterally. That is truly an expression of pleasure. Another muscle, the levator anguli oris—the one that forms an expression of confidence—will also be covered. It would be an aid to the self-image and probably good business as well, to keep that one clear of spasm. All those muscles will be pressed as you move along line A.

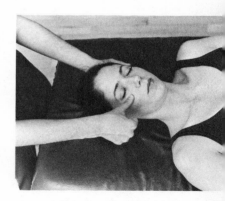

The top of the cheekbone must also be checked, this time by pressing down on the ridge of the bone. Follow the same line A, but about one half inch above it. Do both sides of the face. Stretch by moving the cheeks in several directions.

TRIGGER POINT ERASURE AROUND THE EARS

Start at line B at the outside edge of the eye (see Plate 15 in Appendix 1), and using either the knuckle or the fingers, head for the curve of the ear. This area is almost always sensitive. As

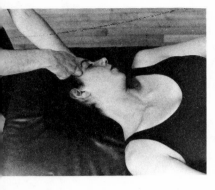

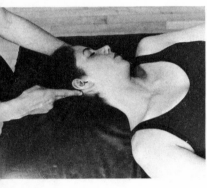

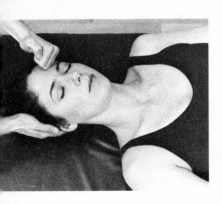

we press along line B at half-inch intervals we go over the temporalis muscles (see Plate 14) which have the job of closing the jaws. That sounds both useful and uncomplicated unless you tend to tighten your jaws when under pressure. Later we will discuss TMJD (temporomandibular joint dysfunction, a jaw pain) in which these muscles are implicated.

Another important muscle, the temporoparietalis, tightens the scalp and if you are sometimes aware that your scalp feels like a too-tight helmet, there are probably trigger points in this area. You will cover it as you approach the ear and later on Line C. Don't worry about finding the muscles—just find the sore and sensitive spots and clear them.

Next is line C, shown on Plate 15, which is a circle rather than a straight line. Press at half-inch intervals all the way around the ear, holding for five seconds when you hit a trigger point. At the back of the ear you will encounter the posterior auricular muscle, which draws the ear backward. I learned when I was a teenager and forced to sit long hours in chapel with a veil bobby-pinned to my hair, that if I could get this muscle going I could wag that veil back and forth and even wiggle my ears. This area also seems to be responsible at least in part for tinnitus, a ringing or buzzing in the ears.

Still on the line-C circle and progressing downward, you will come to the sternocleidomastoid, probably the most important of the lot. Look at Plates 14 and 15 and note that one attachment is at the mastoid process in the skull (spot 65 on Plate 15). From that point, the muscle descends down over the neck to attach to both the sternum (breastbone), spot 73, and the clavicle (collarbone), spot 74, both on Plate 14. In a little while you will learn of the enormous importance of these two muscles in such problems as dizziness and referred pain in the ears, eyes, teeth, and elsewhere. At this moment we are concerned only with the part that attaches to the mastoid process and is on the line-C circle. Continue pressing at half-inch intervals until you have gone full circle. Repeat for the other ear.

Grid A, as shown on Plate 12, is neither a line nor a circle but a field for quartering. Use the roller technique with your knuckles, stopping every four or five spots to stretch the scalp.

Starting around the head toward the back you come to the temporalis, grid B on Plate 14. This area seems to be the primary seat of the "migraine" headache. Looking at grid B on the drawing, you can understand the derivation of the word *migraine*, which means "half head."

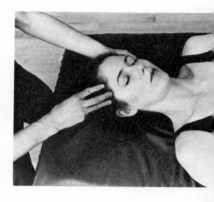

Press three fingers against the temporalis area in grid B and move the scalp in small circles. If a painful spot is found, hold the pressure over it for five seconds and move all three fingers slightly to another spot on the grid. Stretch the scalp every four or five trigger points. Do both sides and proceed to the back of the head.

Along about now, you are probably wondering how much more there is to do. I didn't say this work was going to be quick, only that it works 95 percent of the time. Have heart. You now have only the back of the head to do.

It is helpful if your subject had a headache when you started, so that at this point you can ask him or her to sit up and tell you what spot now houses the pain. *If the subject says the spot has moved, you have it made.* We have found that if the pain responds by shifting to another area on the head, it invariably gives way sooner or later. When we asked Craig, the child of the forehead bump, where it had gone to, he said variously, "Behind my eye," or "To my neck," or at one time, "Would you believe, in my nose?" We believed. His pain was chased from his neck to his shoulders to his back, right down to his left heel. If a long second toe can cause headache (see under The Classic Greek Foot in Chapter 6), there is no reason why a headache cannot, by whatever strange chain of command, cause leg cramps. Usually by the time you get to the back of the head, the ache will have shifted two or three times—if it hasn't left altogether.

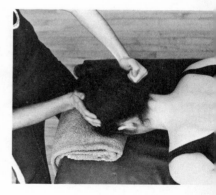

Have the subject lie prone, head resting on the hands or on a folded towel. The face is straight down and the nose protected. The best tools are the knuckles and fingers. The area to be covered is grid C on Plate 13. The muscles are the occipitals.

A trigger point anywhere in the head can refer pain to the back of the head via something with a beautiful name, the galea aponeurotica. *Galea* means "helmet," and an aponeurosis is a white, flattened or ribbonlike tendinous expansion which usually connects muscles with the parts they move. In this case it connects the muscles in the front of the head with those in the back of the head. Pain doesn't go through your head, the way it feels, nor is it inside your head. Pain moves over your head and is, in 95 percent of the headaches, on your head.

55

Proceed to press with fingers or knuckles along line D (see Plate 13) at the base of grid C, from one side back of the ear to the other. Then using the roller technique, cover grid C.

TEMPOROMANDIBULAR JOINT DYSFUNCTION—A PAIN IN THE JAW

This next section is not separate from the material on the head; it is a part of it and would logically be the next step in "head hunting." But the problem of jaw pain has become so prevalent it should be discussed before we go further so you will understand why, with headache, we take in the face, jaw, neck, chest, and shoulders—and why in jaw pain we cover every inch of the head.

TMJD is a problem that until a few years ago did not even have a name. That's because it has so many symptoms that are similar to those of other diseases. As a result, just about every type of medical professional is consulted. Now, however, it is getting enormous attention, and there is even a specialty within a specialty and a professional association for its practitioners, the American Academy of Cranial Mandibular Orthopedics—*cranial* referring to the head; *mandibular* to the jaw. We have already covered the head part of the subspecialty. The jaw part is coming up.

Medical and dental communities are divided over what causes TMJD and just as divided on what to do about it. It is a condition about which you need to be informed, especially if you are a woman (and most TMJD sufferers are women), lest you fall between two points of view.

First, where is it? The name temporomandibular joint dysfunction looks formidable, but as usual medical expertise locates the condition precisely. *Temporo* refers to the temporal bone in the skull. *Mandibular* refers to the mandible, or jawbone. Put those two bones together, and you have a joint. Add a problem and you get dysfunction. So much for where it is. Now, how does it work?

The top of the mandible (jawbone) is ball shaped and fits into the hollow area in the temporal bone on the side of the skull. There is a small disc that separates the two body parts. The entire joint is sheathed in supporting ligaments. When the mouth is opened or closed the mandible moves and is controlled by powerful antigravity muscles (the masseters and pterygoids), which can move it up or down and, to a lesser degree, sideways.

Now, What Is TMJD?

Let's listen to Dr. Janet Travell on the subject:

"Involuntary shortening of one or more of the masticatory muscles may cause an eccentric position of the mandibular condyle [joint], disorientation of jaw movements and restricted opening of the mouth. Also, clicking and grating sounds can be created by abnormal tensions in the muscles that cross the temporomandibular joint and bind its articular surfaces together. Pain is the outstanding complaint."

Temporomandibular joint movement is unique in that any movement of one side depends on appropriate cooperation from the paired joint on the other side. Remember that fact, for it has enormous importance where myotherapy and the relief of pain from TMJD is concerned, for if there are trigger points in one side of the jaw, there will be trigger points in the other side as well, and they must be extinguished, too.

When we talk about taking spasm out of damaged muscles, the question arises as to whether that spasm isn't in the muscle for our protection. The answer is that at first the shortening of a muscle under stress represents the body's effort to protect itself against injury. According to Dr. Travell, "The protective splinting [shortening] . . . tends to gain momentum so that increasing numbers of related groups develop spasm and the pathways of the spasm-pain-spasm chain reaction become extensively facilitated. As a result, painful spasm and its concomitants outlast the precipitating event, and the passage of time does not bring about recovery. Injury initiates a deteriorative biochemical cycle."

The jaw area abounds in trigger points just waiting for the right "climate." Notice that the head, with its many muscles and repeated injuries is not merely close by, it is actually part of the joint. Even something as seemingly unimportant as bumping your head against another's can have disastrous consequences. The vulnerable neck is the joint's nearest neighbor and the neck is supported by the shoulders, over which are draped the usually tense trapezius muscles. The shoulders are attached to the arms and hands, which themselves are often damaged by trauma.

57

In addition to such dangerous neighbors, the jaw houses within its very walls a potentially troublesome fifth column, teeth. Teeth are usually good citizens unless infected, at which time they can refer pain to their host, the jaw. If a tooth has the temerity to grow too tall, or in the wrong direction, then the tooth itself can cause malocclusion (poor bite), the condition responsible for at least a goodly number of TMJD cases.

The nasal and paranasal cavities are to the TMJ like folks sharing a two-family house. One need not ever hear from the other as long as all is well, but a fire in one could put a pox on both apartments.

Also, the temporomandibular joint is within 2 or 3 millimeters of the inner ear. They too can live in harmony, or they can exchange pain. Earache is a common symptom in TMJD. By the same token, jaw pain and limitation of movement can cause pain to settle in the ear. Neighboring structures should always be treated as suspect in any joint pain.

In the absence of pathology, TMJD exhibits multiple signals which add up to nothing you can pin a tail to. Like the chronic back sufferer, the TMJD patient will also go the medical rounds. The symptoms sound like a hypochondriac's nightmare, and which way the arrow points merely depends on which symptom surfaces first.

One evening at a cocktail party one of our young myotherapists was told by a friend that she had just had a root canal job done. She was thinking it must have been the wrong tooth because there was still just as much pain in her lower jaw as before. The next day she was slated for another root canal. The myotherapist asked her where the pain started. In her neck she said. The myotherapist set to work, the party forgotten. One hour later the neck was relaxed, the pain gone from the jaw and mouth, and the appointment card torn up. That was two years ago, and the pain has not returned.

The nature of the onset of TMJD, like its symptoms, varies. It can come on quite suddenly. Usually it is brought on by some traumatic episode such as a blow to the face or a too forcible tooth extraction, especially an impacted third molar. Clicking and limitation of jaw motion may follow singly or to-together. As in other kinds of pain involving trigger points, muscles gradually shorten under tonic spasm. Even when the onset is sudden, the stage was probably set long before when the muscles were insulted.

Because of the interdependence of the two sides of the mandible, many doctors and dentists (but not all by any means) believe that as many as 90 percent of all TMJD cases are the result of malocclusion. It is quite true that jaw pain can sometimes be caused by an occlusal imbalance, and it is also true that it can be caused by an infected tooth or a respiratory infection. But far more often I believe, it is due to the terrible trio—trigger point, tension, and triggering mechanism.

A very revealing statistic was provided recently on the numbers and sexes of people suffering with TMJD. There are said to be 4 million sufferers in this country and that of those, 3.8 million are women. Why does this problem strike women so much more frequently than men? My theory is that since men have as many under- and overshot jaws as women, just as good or bad teeth as women, just as good or poor bites as women, there has to be something else. There is: frustration.

Let's do an experiment; find the masseter. The masseter is king muscle in the jaw. Place your fingers on each side of your face just in front of your earlobes. Relax your jaws completely. Now, clench your teeth, hard. The lumps rising from your jaws are the masseters. What do you do when you are angry but can't let it out? You clamp your jaws tight. What do you do when you want and need to cry, but you can't? You clamp your jaws tight. What do you do when your dreams are filled with situations you can't resolve? You clamp your jaws tight. What causes most jaw pain? Again, I think it must be the terrible trio—trigger points, tension, and triggering mechanism, with emphasis on tension, this time in the form of frustration. Check your bed again. True, you may have made it, but do you have to lie there with a pain in your jaw? Is there also a pain in your heart?

One clinic, where 350 TMJD patients are treated yearly, reports that 300 of that number are women. It is claimed that "Certain personality types, like the up-tight housewife who may or may not have *real* (italics mine) problems, are the major sufferers." However, with or without *real* problems, six or seven patients a year are given surgery; the others treated with medications, mouth splints, injections, and advice on how to relax their jaw.

Many dentists put their faith in the plastic appliances designed to correct malocclusion. While some do not believe in their value, others make them the basis of their practice. One patient who was sent to our institute hoping myotherapy would

59

help, had had just such a gadget locked in her mouth by the spasm that followed its insertion. It had been imprisoned for almost a year. It was fortunate in one way that her diet was almost totally liquid, because in addition to her TMJD she had another problem, nausea and vomiting through her nose.

In addition to the plastic appliances there are splints, braces, procaine and Xylocaine injections, and steroid injections. Critics hold that this last is not in the best interest of the patient, since steroids are said to destroy brain tissue and may even cause brain abscesses. The jaw isn't all that far from the brain.

There is of course the usual list of palliatives: hot packs, cold packs, diathermy and massage, or a diet limited to soft or semisoft food for months on end. One dentist insists that his patients make an effort to limit the extent of mouth opening even when laughing or yawning. They are told to cut all food into small pieces and avoid any foods that require excessive chewing. That's like confining a weak leg in a brace in order not to overtax it. What the jaw needs is not a brace, but to be free of the trigger points causing the spasm that is resulting in both pain and malocclusion.

Research of the last 30 years indicates that most of the complaints leading to TMJD are attributed to what Dr. Travell calls myofascial-pain-dysfunction syndrome and what we call trigger points. The next question is, what can we do about it?

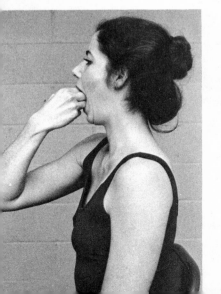

JAW PAIN PLUS HEAD PAIN (CONTINUED)

First, have the subject see how many knuckles will fit in the mouth. Three seems to be normal, but the person who has suffered a jaw or head injury often has trouble getting the mouth wide enough for two.

The place to start for the jaw pain is where we left off, in the back of the head. You covered line D (see Plate 13). In line D are two circles numbered 66. These are exceptionally important as well as usually painful. Under those circles are crossroads where several powerful and often overused muscles come together. The splenius capitis (see Plates 13 and 14), semispinalis capitis, and the upper reaches of the trapezius, that huge capelike muscle which is draped over very tense shoulders: all those muscles converge under spot 66.

Using either your finger or your knuckle, press upward into the curve of the skull, the occipital bone, in the little hollow off to the side of the neck.

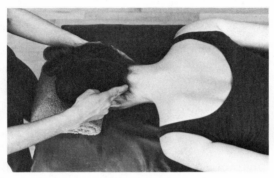

The splenius attaches to the cervical vertebrae in the neck and the three upper thoracic (chest) vertebrae in the upper back. Refer to Plate 14 and you will see three circles labeled 70, 71, and 72. Those three look as if they were on the trapezius, and they are, but under the trapezius lies the splenius, traveling downward.

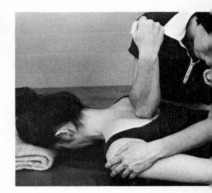

Use your finger or knuckle and press in each of those circles. Do both sides. You have now hit the upper attachment of the splenius and the upper attachment of the trapezius, but you still need the lower attachment of the splenius. Refer to Plate 5 in Appendix 1. Spot 18 is where you will find the attachment, and if your subject has frequent headaches, stiff necks, or shoulder pain, it will be sensitive indeed. Use the elbow for this muscle and having found one sensitive spot, search around for a few more. Do both sides.

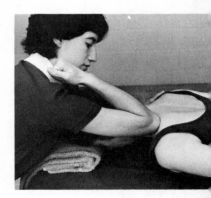

Next the trapezius should be checked at the shoulder, both front and back. Stand at the head of the table and press your elbow straight into the top of the shoulder. Go back to holding the pressure for seven seconds. Do both sides.

To get at the front side of the trapezius, move to the side of the table and change tools from elbow to fingers. Using the fingers of one hand to reach into the soft triangle in front of that muscle, and the fingers of the other hand to cover and give power, pull back. Hold for seven seconds and do the other side. If this area is extremely sensitive use the Double Massage suggested on page 132 often.

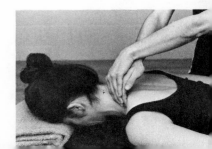

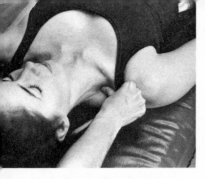

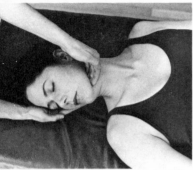

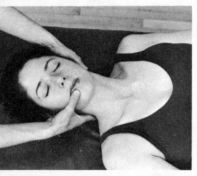

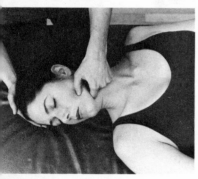

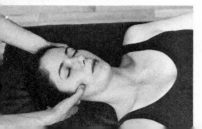

People who have jobs that involve the shoulders damage them in small ways constantly. Microtrauma results from small repetitive motions.

The scalene muscles (see Plate 14) are found by pressing the thumb into the triangular space back of the clavicle (collarbone). That search too calls for moving the tool (the thumb) in several directions searching for sore spots.

The platysma, shown in Plate 15, is a "weak" muscle which we share with other animals. Fortunately, it is more than a little weak in alligators, which is why their trainers, the people who for whatever reason wrestle alligators, can clamp their jaws tight and keep them that way. Weak or strong, if a platysma harbors trigger points they can affect both jaw and head. Turn the head to the side and press up against the underside of the jaw from ear to ear at half-inch intervals. This technique involves using the flat of the hand.

The orbicularis oris (Plate 12) circles the mouth, and if one side of your mouth tends to droop, check this muscle. Start at one side of the lower lip and using either finger or thumb, circle the entire mouth at half-inch intervals.

Now for the upper side of the jaw. Using the thumb on top of the jawbone and a curved index finger, move from the point of the jaw to the ear on both sides. Keep to the half-inch intervals.

Now we come to the king pin, the masseter. Trigger points in one part of this muscle can cause pain in the molars of the upper jaw; in another part, the pain would appear in the lower molars.

Have the subject relax his or her jaw so the teeth do not touch. Using your thumb, press backward on the leading edge of the muscle. This will be sensitive in almost everyone, but for the person with TMJD it could feel like a crisis. Don't cause more pain than the subject can take without tensing, and when you let up, massage the muscle with your thumb before going on. Use two fingers against the back edge of the masseter and follow with massage. The stretch for this muscle is opening the mouth wide. If the subject's jaw is afflicted with the tendency to subluxate (slip partially out of joint, or feel as though it were) the masseter is probably in spasm. If you can't get more than two knuckles into your mouth, the masseter is probably in spasm. Let's go on to the neck.

TRIGGER POINT ERASURE AROUND THE NECK

My father-in-law used to smile as he said, "Yes, I'm the head of the house, but my wife is the neck that turns the head." My mother-in-law used to smile too—because it was true. The neck does turn the head—or refuses to. It houses the magic strings that pour forth logic, vituperation, and song—or, muted by disease, remain silent. The neck supports the head proudly, tilts it saucily, or droops it in sad dejection. The neck provides the head and body with the opportunity to express a thousand moods and nuances.

On a different note, the neck holds the secret to most dizziness. Little kids turn round and round to get themselves dizzy. Then they fall on the grass and watch the clouds lurch around the sky. Big kids keep on drinking beer until some of them fall flat and watch the others lurch around the room. Those two dizzies are harmless enough. One gets over them, and those kids know how they got dizzy in the first place.

Last month as I was doing some TV spots around the country talking about myotherapy, the interviewer brought up the subject of dizziness. She said she wished there were a trigger point for dizziness, but alas, she had hypoglycemia, and whenever she moved her head quickly or leaned over she felt as though she would fall flat.

I said, "Like a kid that has the dizzies from turning round and round?" Yes, that was exactly how she felt. I asked if she'd been given the glucose test for hypoglycemia and found out that no, she hadn't. Who then had diagnosed her ailment? She (like at least 50 million of us) had read about it in a magazine.

Her hypoglycemia was gone in less than three minutes when I cleared the trigger points from both sternocleidomastoids. She went around bending over and shaking her head and feeling younger and better every minute.

There is still another kind of dizziness, a condition you don't have but might get. During last week's lunch with my mother-in-law, when her little tray of medicines was brought for her unquestioning consumption, I gleaned this little bit of education.

"What's that one for?" asked the heretic, me.

"That's an antivertigo medication," said her companion.

"Has she got vertigo?"

"No, but we don't want her to get it."

63

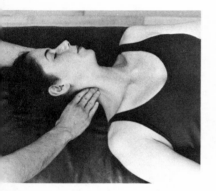

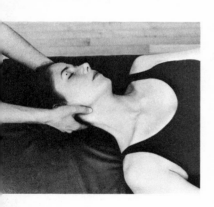

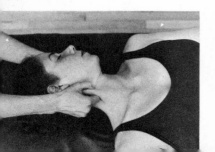

Dizziness can be caused by many things. Before ascribing it to disease, clear the sternocleidomastoids and the other trigger point havens in the head. Then, if the subject's gait is still like that of Captain Ahab ashore, think pathological.

A final word on dizziness. Don't assign magazine diseases to yourself. Start reading some books on medical history and see how many diseases have been "discovered" that nobody ever really had. Sufficient unto the day is the evil thereof—don't add unfounded fears to compound it.

The sternocleidomastoid has a formidable name. If you know what its parts stand for, however, it's as easy as any other three-part name, say John Q. Public. *Sterno* stands for the sternum, or breastbone, where one of its attachments is. The muscle has two heads: *cleido* stands for the clavicle, or collarbone, where a second attachment is found; *mastoid* is for the mastoid process behind the ear where the upper attachment is. Simple and beautifully logical.

Something else could be beautifully logical. The girl who broke her collarbone falling off her horse at the show develops TMJD, or "migraines." None of the conventional medications works, nor do mouth splints. The continued diagnostic search may well dig up the cause: trigger points somewhere in the sterno-cleido-mastoid.

We have already touched on the upper attachment of the SCM when we went around the ear on line C (see Plate 15, spot 65). Now we plan to erase trigger points all along its length. Start with the subject lying supine, head turned to the side, which brings the muscle into view.

Use three fingers to press against the back edge of the muscle and work toward the belly of the muscle, a spot that most people find tender. Almost anyone who has ever had a whiplash will cringe. Then, using the thumb, press toward the belly of the muscle on the leading, or front, edge.

When you have cleared those two points, change your technique. Apply the "squeeze." This must be done gently until most of the trigger points have been investigated at least twice.

Tip the subject's head sideways and down toward your working hand and grasp the relaxed muscle between the thumb and bent forefinger. Bring the head back so the subject faces the ceiling and work your way down to the sternum at half-inch intervals. Check out the two lower attachments to the sternum and clavicle at spots 73 and 74 as shown on Plate 6 in Appendix 1. Do both sides.

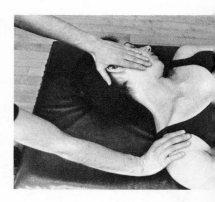

To stretch the muscles after clearing trigger points, turn the subject's head to the side while anchoring the opposite shoulder against the table. Hold the stretch a few seconds, release, and repeat three more times.

Behind the sternocleidomastoid are several vulnerable and important muscles. We have already met the splenius capitis, but there is also the levator scapulae, which is involved in shoulder tension. The scalene muscles have similar properties. Check Plate 14 for positions of these muscles.

Start near the base of the skull and, using all four fingers, move down just behind the sternocleidomastoid at half-inch intervals, pressing first toward the muscle and then away. (The first illustration in this section shows where to work.) *Do both sides.*

STRETCH AND RESISTANCE EXERCISE FOR NECK

Your subject has had most of the neck, face, and head muscles cleared, and now the muscles need both stretch and resistance.

Have him or her sit in a chair while you stand behind it. Place your hands on either side of the subject's face as though placing blinders on a horse. Turn the head as far to the left as possible, instructing the subject to note what can be seen at the extreme view. Do the same to the right. Next, place your palms against both cheeks and have the subject turn the head from right to left and left to right in a slow rhythm.

Remove one hand and gradually apply a little pressure with the hand remaining to provide resistance saying, "Just push my hand as you turn your head." Alternating hands, do four turns from side to side.

Now place your hand under the subject's chin, asking him to press his chin downward and look into his lap as you apply resistance. While the subject's head is tipped down place your

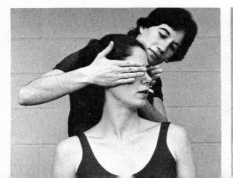
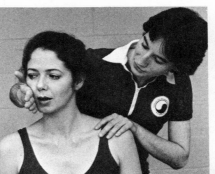
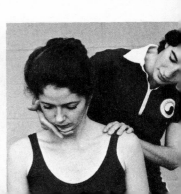

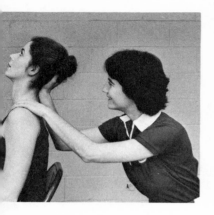

hand across the back of the head and ask the subject to tip the head backward and look at the ceiling. Do four of these, up and down, with resistance. If you have the coolant spray, this is a good time to use it, spraying along any muscle that is either tight or painful—spray *as* you stretch. (See under Immediate Mobilization in Chapter 7.)

Alternate four times left and right and four times up and down.

After these resistance exercises are finished, try again with "blinders" to check how much farther the subject can see to the left and right. Unless he or she was just about perfect to begin with, there will be increased range.

You have completed your first go-round with head, face, and neck. If your subject has less pain or no pain, you are a success. Remember, however, that if you overlooked any satellites (and you probably did, because often they are in the second or third layer of armoring), the matrix points may light up again. Again, take heart. You will find them next time or the time after next. If the injury causing the pain occurred yesterday or last week, relief will be quick. If it was long ago, it will take a little longer. The exercises, the neck resistance you just did, the shrugs (page 99), and the shoulder rotations (page 122), will be helpful when done daily.

Americans are bombarded with stimuli and very few of us have sufficient physical outlet to balance them out. Whatever we do that is physical usually adds more tension to shoulders and neck and, therefore, head. We jog, we play tennis, we play golf, we bowl, all of which cause tension in those areas if we don't use counteracting exercise. Combining our occupations and our pleasures adds up to lots of pressure on the back of the neck and on the head and shoulders. These have to be booby-trap-alley, nowhere for a healthy muscle to live.

Arthritis Pain Can Be Relieved

6

I could not count the number of people who come to the institute for work on "arthritis of the spine," "an arthritic knee," "arthritis in the fingers, wrist, elbow, shoulder, ankles, feet."

ARTHRITIS STRIKES NEARLY EVERYONE

As it happens, only 50 percent of the people with arthritis suffer any symptoms of the disease. For example, many who have arthritis of the spine find out only when they are X-rayed for something else, an injury, or an acute back spasm, for example. It is then that they learn the awful truth, they have arthritis of the spine. Sure they have it, and so do most others over 45. But what doesn't bother, doesn't call for X-ray, so they have never seen the evidence of their arthritis.

Arthritis isn't the cause of the pain in most cases. Back muscles in spasm cause the pain. Erase the pain by erasing the trigger points, and the arthritis isn't a terrifier anymore.

At this point we are not talking about rheumatoid arthritis, which we will get to later. Now we are discussing plain old every day osteoarthritis. The Greeks, as usual, had the necessary words, *osteon* meaning "bone" and *arthron* meaning "joint" plus *itis* for "inflammation." That's the kind that just about everybody has a "touch" of—or expects to.

Osteoarthritis has a history that reaches back into the far distant past. Animals roaming the earth six million years ago had it, as did the Stone Age people. Ape man had it and so did Ape woman two million years ago. Java man and Neanderthal Man and their mates had it and so did the Egyptians who came along about ten thousand years later. The Greeks and the Romans were not exempt (nor had their physician-priests found any way to prevent or cure it). The Vandals and the Goths trampled the civilized world under arthritic feet, and the blue-painted inhabitants of the British Isles must have had their full share since arthritis thrives in wet, cold climates. All those many wars they fought could not have been of much help either, since arthritis rides in on the heels of wounds and is tied to the tail of fever.

The U.S. Census Bureau states that there are twenty million Americans suffering with arthritis and that one out of every ten people have some form of it. They claim that ten million have osteo and six million rheumatoid. But the Census Bureau gets its information from the people, many of whom don't know they have arthritis (50 percent have no symptoms, remember). The specialists in arthritis clinics all over the country say there are more than forty million with osteo alone. That disease usually hits people over forty. Since there are about sixty million in this country in that age bracket, that would mean that two out of every three have osteo—or the condition that feels like it, myofascial (muscular) pain.

In the short twenty years between ages forty and sixty, arthritis in one of its forms will begin to attack 97 percent of the population. To death and taxes one should really add arthritis. Nearly 100 percent of all people over sixty-five are said to show arthritic changes which are picked up by X-ray. Fortunately, only half those people suffer pain, swelling, or loss of range and coordination. While you are reading these ominous statistics, remember that trigger points also cause pain, swelling, and loss of range and coordination, and you already know how to deal with those.

Osteo affects both men and women equally, though men seem to have it more often in the lumbar spine, probably because their sports and their occupations require greater effort. Women are not usually as active in a physically destructive way, and when they are overactive, as in childbirth, the stress is limited to hours. Men's physical stresses often last a lifetime.

When the longshoreman goes to the company doctor with back pain and the X-rays show arthritis (and they most likely will whether the arthritis is the cause of the pain or not), he will be told he has no anatomic pathology, that the X-rays show only a little old arthritis, and that he should give up lifting. It's easy for the doctor to deliver those words, not so easy for the patient to follow them. What else can he do to make a living? The next steps will be all downhill, as he goes the backache round at the expense of the insurance company that handles his union policy.

HAPPILY, ARTHRITIS PAIN RESPONDS TO MYOTHERAPY

You know, however, that arthritis can lay down trigger points in muscles and that old traumas leave footprints all over the body in which arthritis is delighted to follow. The saving grace? The pain caused by arthritis does respond to myotherapy.

It is thought that osteoarthritis is related to age and weight and in all probability the two in tandem. We would add another cause—damage. Any damage done to the body attracts arthritis. The longer you live, the more time you have for attracting damage, great or small. Arthritis is not caused by age per se. If there is no pain or weakness in the body, and if the blood vessels are free to do their work efficiently, unimpeded by constricting muscle spasms caused by trigger points laid down over the years, then age just doesn't matter.

SPLINTING AND SUBSTITUTION

The longer the trigger points related to arthritis go unattended, however, the more time the muscles have in which to learn bad habits. Two of the bad habits are called splinting, or guarding, and substitution. Splinting is a shortening of the muscle into spasms in an attempt to guard against pain. Eventually, the shortening of those muscles protecting the body with spasm becomes chronic; the muscles actually lose their ability to relax, and their tonic (constant) spasm exhausts the sufferer even when the pain is kept at bay by medication. Muscles are terrible slaves to habit, and if the habit of splinting is in force long enough, it's very hard to break.

The other bad habit, substitution, was once presented to me as "a delicate art." The muscles are hurt, and they cannot

69

move as they were meant to, and they cannot do the work for which they were designed, so we substitute other muscles, muscles not designed for that job or not capable of handling two jobs. Then we get into another kind of trouble. We develop the habit, say, of walking on the outside edge of a foot that was sprained. Nothing was done about the sprain, of course, other than taping, resting, heat, cold, and arnica. Pretty soon the knee begins to ache, then the hip, then the back.

Dizzy Dean, the famous baseball pitcher, learned first-hand about the dangers of substitution. One day, Dizzy injured his foot. Ignoring the hurt, he went on pitching using an unnatural pitching motion. The result: By favoring his foot, he ruined his arm and ended a spectacular career.

This is something for you to keep in mind: A small pain can lead to a bigger one. All pains should be considered serious and erased at once with myotherapy. This prevents bad muscular habits which lead to worse problems, more pain, and, sometimes, arthritis. The longshoreman with a backache is an "idler"—without one he is a longshoreman again.

PREVALENCE OF ARTHRITIS BY OCCUPATION

Arthritis is more prevalent in rural areas than in cities. More of our farmers have it than our professional and technical workers. I found no statistics on farmers' wives (or any other wives for that matter) so I will assume it is the job rather than the location that is the cause.

There is more arthritis in lower income groups. That would certainly bear out the theory that hard work and a high level of emotional stress combine disastrously. My mother, who had a saying for everything, always remarked when my sister or I brought home a boy with no visible means of support, "When poverty flies in the window, love flies out the door." I'd change that to read, "When poverty and its attendants, overwork and anxiety, stalk in the door, it's an invitation to arthritis—whether love stays home or not."

There is more arthritis in the damp, cold Northeast than anywhere else in the country. Now, that might be worth knowing if you are thinking of retiring and something hurts. Even if no one has suggested your hurt might be arthritis, it might be a good idea to investigate the more comfortable Southwest. Arizona and New Mexico have the lowest incidence of arthritis of all the states.

Look at the following selection of types of workers listed in descending order according to the incidence of arthritis in each type. Ask yourself what part emotional stress may have played in triggering the disease and in maintaining its destructive progress.

Incidence of Arthritis Among Various Types of Workers, in Descending Order of Occurrence

1. Farmers. They are overworked and their crops depend on a very uncertain factor—weather. Lots of stress.
2. Factory workers. Many are bored to death and often physically stressed by repetitious movement or limited movement.
3. Craftsmen and foremen. Their jobs demand both concentration and responsibility. Foremen must direct others and are responsible for the quality of work. This contributes to anxiety, frustration, and often anger.
4. Managers, store owners, and company officials. This group has less than half the arthritis suffered by farmers, but double that of lawyers, doctors, and technicians. Since the physical work is not extreme, the stress of responsibility is at the root of the problem. For company officials it may well be the rat race known as competition.
5. Construction. Construction workers usually do heavy work, but their physical activity helps to relieve stress.
6. Wholesale and retail workers. It's hard to say why they are in the middle ground. There is often a great deal of stress connected with dealing with the public. There is responsibility in buying and selling, but perhaps the fact that physical strain is absent may be a plus.
7. Finance, insurance, real estate workers. Responsibility within bounds, and they are usually self-employed. Ample opportunity to get out of the office is available to them.
8. Service workers. No real responsibility, plus at least some opportunity for physical release.
9. Clerical. Responsibility usually assumed by someone else. Prime danger is lack of physical activity, which does not

seem as damaging as overactivity. In this case the heart is more at risk than joints.

10. Transportation and public utilities. Again the responsibility is someone else's. For those who drive, the heart is at risk and the back pain is usually from trigger points in muscles.

11. Laborers other than farm workers. No real responsibility is involved. Their low arthritis rate would make it seem that mental stress has more to do with arthritis than physical exertion.

12. Professional and technical workers. Since doctors have a high heart attack rate it looks as though there might be something to the phrase, "Get arthritis and your heart is safe." If you had to choose, I'd say settle for arthritis; we can keep that pain under control.

13. Salesworkers. The job is nine to five and the manager has the responsibility.

14. Private household workers. Today, hours are reasonably short. In addition, appliances make easy work of household chores. A certain amount of physical activity offsets any stress present.

THE TYPES OF ARTHRITIS

There is unquestionably a relationship between arthritis and some heavy labor, but there is an even stronger relationship between arthritis and emotional stress. Most people can trace the onset of the disease, or at least the first appearance of symptoms, to an incident or sequence of events that affected them deeply.

If you have true arthritis or suffer from myofascial pain, which feels as though it ought to be arthritis, you have lots of company. In many cases osteoarthritis is age-related, since older people have had more time for wear and tear to do their work.

It is now believed that there are four common forms of arthritis: osteoarthritis, rheumatoid arthritis, gouty arthritis, and infectious arthritis. It is also thought that arthritis may result from any one of 150 odd diseases from which man and woman suffer, often without knowing it, and often without diagnosis or treatment of the disease.

Osteoarthritis

Osteoarthritis causes progressive degeneration of the cartilage in a joint. It is associated with wear and tear and is often considered to be a part of the aging process. However, it attacks young people too when there is excessive wear through sports or heavy labor. There are two basic types, primary and secondary. Primary osteoarthritis is the type in which there is gradual degeneration of what was once a healthy joint. The cause is not completely known. Heredity, heavy work loads, and obesity are all said to be involved.

Secondary osteoarthritis is due to a specific cause such as an injury to the joint, some mechanical imbalance (such as one leg shorter than the other), or a congenital anomaly. The injury could be massive, as was the pelvic fracture that led to both my hip joints being replaced. Or it could be the result of many small, repeated injuries such as those suffered by athletes, especially runners. While the causes differ, the degenerative process is the same in both types.

As the cartilage is gradually destroyed, the raw surface of the underlying bone is exposed and becomes exquisitely tender. The pain can be excruciating. Articular cartilage cannot regenerate itself, so the body in a desperate effort to repair the damage replaces it with bone. Unfortunately, it doesn't know when to stop. This results in knobby enlargements of the joints. The second and third joints of the fingers are a well-known battleground for osteo. If you have painful knobbies, follow the instructions in Chapter 7 (see under The Hand) on erasing hand pain. If you have painful fingers and hands without knobbies, think myofascial pain, usually referred from somewhere else higher up. The same trigger points will be involved; only the cause is different.

In osteoarthritis, a primary characteristic is the development of bony spurs around the arthritic joint. Now the very word *spur* makes one think of sharp spikes, and if there is pain in the area of the spurs, we may imagine them digging into the quivering flesh. This may cause us to exaggerate a limp, or, in the case of "cervical spurs," further immobilize the head and neck.

I had one woman sent to me wearing one of those miserable neck collars. She had headache and back pain, and her neck was "full of bony spurs." "The doctor told me if I moved my head quickly I could cut my spinal cord and I'd be a quadriplegic," she told me. Now there's food for nightmares. It took roughly half an hour to talk about the real problem, trigger points in her neck and shoulders. By applying the appropriate myotherapy technique (instructions for which you will find in the appropriate chapters in this book), it took even less time than that to get rid of her headache, stiff neck, and back pain.

One of the problems we have in taking care of our bodies is that we know so little about them. When bone spurs are mentioned we visualize pointy spikes, such as those used for climbing a pole. We should, in fact, picture the short, stunted branches of a tree. There is no rule that says a spur of land has to have a point on it, is there? Well, the spurs you pick up through injury or disease are apt to be round and lumpy, and the pain you feel is far more often due to trigger points causing muscle spasm than a large pointed thorn which "could cut your spinal cord."

Rheumatoid Arthritis

Rheumatoid arthritis is something else again. Not content to confine its depredations to joints, it invades the whole body system. It moves in for years and sometimes for always. It can take a vacation called remission, but it's usually only a vacation. The host may think the problem has gone for good. Not so. It can move back at any time and in any intensity. Intensity can range from a few "arthritic" aches and pains to a raging inflammation consuming the entire body.

Rheumatoid usually starts with an acute inflammation of the synovial membrane within a joint. The job of the synovial membrane is to lubricate the joint and provide smooth, painfree function. When rheumatoid goes to work there are many unpleasant changes, among them swelling from the excessive accumulation of fluid. The synovial lining thickens and overgrows. The joint enlarges and ligaments are stretched, which weakens the joint and interferes with its function. Eventually the auricular cartilage is completely destroyed. This inflammatory process is unbearably painful, and this causes the sufferer to stop moving the affected joint, which results in more destructive changes. In addition, trigger points are laid down in the muscles surrounding the joint as well as those far distant from ground zero.

The trigger points accompanying osteoarthritis can be extinguished any time, but those connected with the arthritis of the rheumatoid sufferer must wait until any period of severe inflammation is past. Myotherapy can erase the trigger points for both conditions, but if the diseased joint puts out noxious feedback, the trigger points will be influenced to light up again. This means that the work will have to be done for some people on a continuing basis.

Myotherapy cannot "cure" arthritis, but it can reduce and often erase the pain in the spasmed muscles which pull on the joints. By relaxing the spasm, myotherapy can increase the nutrition of the joint, which can promote healing. Vessels, cramped by the viselike pressure of the muscles in tonic spasm, cannot deliver a good blood supply to an afflicted area. If myotherapy is used on a continuing basis, pain and swelling can be kept to a minimum. Since arthritis is thought to be stress-related, keeping the sufferer active and independent is of primary importance. Rheumatoid attacks and subsides, attacks and subsides. If the body can be maintained in good condition during remissions, then it is fit and equipped to fight hard if another attack comes. This is quite different from the prospect faced by the sufferer who meets each new attack in a weakened condition, with pain and exhaustion as additional enemies.

Some of the early symptoms of rheumatoid can be found in the patient months and sometimes years before it surfaces under its true name. This has given rise to the belief that there are many diseases that lead to arthritis or perhaps diseases of which arthritis is merely the result.

There are many theories as to the cause of rheumatoid arthritis. One is that it is caused by an abnormal antibody created by the body itself. The body has the ability to produce antibodies to protect itself from disease-causing substances. Those antibodies, while harmful to invaders, do not normally harm the body they are protecting, unless, that is, something goes wrong.

It is thought that for some reason (emotional stress is a prime suspect) the body commences to manufacture antibodies that do harm to the body itself. In other words, the body causes its own arthritis. There is good reason to hold this theory because rheumatoid sufferers have in their blood an antibody-like factor called "the rheumatoid factor." People who do not have the disease do not have the factor.

There is another theory that claims widespread interest, which is that rheumatoid is caused by a virus. The theory holds that a virus invades different joints, and even organs, and then lies dormant until it is triggered by an outside force.

Myotherapy will not cure the disease, but it can make the symptoms much less painful and terrifying and thereby alleviate at least some of the stress that seems to trigger or aggravate it.

Gouty Arthritis

Gout isn't really arthritis at all, but the name persists. While it can strike any joint and is frequently seen in both the ankle and knee, most often it settles for the big toe. Dr. Travell says that the long second toe must invite it, because she has not seen a case of gout in a foot that was not also blessed with that anomaly. It does stand to reason that the poor big toe, forced out of its proper line and sprouting an inflamed and painful bunion, would, with its constant trauma, attract something unpleasant.

If you have a long second toe, it would be wise to take the precaution offered on page 89, the innersole with sponge-rubber circlets. There is something else that helps; go without shoes as much as possible or wear sandals. The barefoot and nearly barefoot state allow the toes to reach out normally and produce good balance, which shoes (including ballet slippers) prevent.

While rheumatoid afflicts three times as many women as men, about 93 percent of gouty arthritis is suffered by men. It seems to run in families and is caused by an inborn defect in the metabolism, the chemical process by which food is converted into *energy*. The defect prevents the proper conversion of purines, which abound in many rich foods and may account for the fact that gout has always been considered a rich man's disease. In the disease, the body produces large amounts of uric acid, far more than can be disposed of through urination. Carried by the blood, deposits of the extra uric acid are trapped in the joints where they crystallize and cause inflammation. It is thought that the formation of crystals is in turn triggered by an injury.

Infectious Arthritis

It was recognized centuries ago that people suffering with infections often developed arthritis. They had not labeled infections as such yet, nor did they know that such diseases were caused by specific organisms, but they did know that people who suffered with the "French Pox," as syphilis was then called, most often developed arthritis. Gonorrhea sufferers also showed arthritic symptoms, as did people with tuberculosis. In time, after researchers had isolated the tuberculosis bacterium and also those causing syphilis, gonorrhea, pneumonia, and typhoid, they found the same bacteria in arthritic joints.

While infectious arthritis is considered a common form of arthritis, it is far less common than it used to be, owing to the discovery of antibiotics which control infectious diseases. Still, infectious arthritis, like the other forms, seems to crank up existing trigger points and is probably capable of laying down additional ones.

A joint's susceptibility to infectious arthritis can be greatly increased by injury to the joint or surgery performed on the joint, and this applies equally to the many joints that make up the spine. Even an injection of medication into the joint may make it more vulnerable. It is more than just possible that an injection of cortisone into your "football knee," "bursitis," or "tennis elbow" could leave you worse off than you are. Older people who have been ill for a long time with one disease or another seem especially prone to infectious arthritis, so with that in mind the prevention of disease should be uppermost in all our thoughts. Lack of exercise is a contributing factor to many diseases, as are overeating, heavy drinking, and smoking. A report issued by Wayne State University holds that most of the diseases that lead to our death are self-induced. That means too that we are, at least in part, responsible for our arthritis.

More than half the people with arthritis are getting no treatment at all. Millions who do seek help are misdiagnosed and receive the wrong treatment. Even osteo and rheumatoid can be confused, and although many types of infectious arthritis can be cured, many are overlooked entirely.

MEDICATION AND ARTHRITIS

Rheumatoid arthritis is often treated with steroids which suppress inflammation but do nothing about the disease. This is not the major failing of steroids, however. Many have dangerous side effects which could end up producing problems worse than the disease. Whenever you are given any medication more complicated than aspirin, be sure to ask if you may consult the PDR (Physicians' Desk Reference). We have one at the institute, which we use to check every medication ever taken by the patients referred to us. Some days I feel I'm dealing in wolf bane, lizards' eyes, and cobra venom. If the doctor prefers that you not see what is in the medication prescribed, look it up at the library.

The subject of medication can get really scary. Recently, I sent for pamphlets on three medications used for arthritis. These medications are often prescribed with no warning to the patient about possible side effects and with no set time limit. Also, there is sometimes no supervision in the form of blood tests. I was fed Indocin for my hip pain. One of our young patients was given prednisone and gold salts, which caused many adverse reactions. By the time he came to us, he had given them both up, preferring the pain to the devastating side effects. By the time I reached Dr. Travell, I was still taking many prescribed medications. She gave them up for me and prescribed vitamins.

The following information on the possible side effects of gold salts is based on material provided by pharmaceuticals companies and from a directory of information about drugs. It is easy for the public to obtain. Of course, not everyone using this drug will suffer the side effects. All the same, the fact that they are possible, even if rare, is eye-opening.

Among the most common reactions is dermatitis, including a skin rash or itching. The most serious form is exfoliative dermatitis (all over peeling and scaling), which may lead to baldness and shedding of nails. Other common side effects are ulcers, sores, or white spots in the mouth or throat. In addition, the tongue or gums may become sore or irritated.

Some of the rare side effects include bloody urine or proteinuria (excess of serum protein in the urine). Diarrhea or colitis, sore throat and fever, and unusual fatigue or weakness have also been reported. Eye problems, including conjunctivitis, iritis, and corneal ulcers, may develop with prolonged use of gold salts.

There may also be allergic and nitritoid reactions to the injection. Flushing, fainting, dizziness, and sweating are the most frequently reported. Other symptoms may include nausea, vomiting, and weakness. More severe but less common is an unusually slow heartbeat or a thickening of the tongue.

Finally, arthralgia (pain in a joint) sometimes occurs a day or two after injection. (Now what were those injections given for? Wasn't it arthritis, inflammation, and pain in joints?)

One of my very first experiences with arthritis was with a charming little woman who had had rheumatoid for years and been terribly damaged by it. She had severe contractures in arms, shoulders, and feet. A friend asked me to see if what we did could help in any way, and I said I'd try. In an hour she felt much looser, had more range, and said the pain had eased considerably. After the second session, she was better still, and at the end of the third session she walked all the way down a long hill and back up without any pain in her legs or feet. We felt that, yes, myotherapy could help in cases of rheumatoid arthritis.

It is our policy not to take any people (whatever the problem) not referred by doctors, and I had just been working around the edges to find out if myotherapy would be at all effective on rheumatoid arthritis. Now we wanted to really get down to cases, so I sent her to a family doctor for referral. Seeing all the damage she had suffered over the years, he sent her to a rheumatologist. She was taken off exercise at once and put on gold salts. It's years now and the gains we made are lost. I wonder what results the gold salts have produced.

The pharmaceuticals houses' listing of potential and rare side effects for the two other drugs often prescribed for arthritis are no more reassuring. Indocin, which I took long enough so I began to look like an alligator with hives, is one. Prednisone, the other, can cause varied and profound metabolic effects and can also modify the body's immune response to serious stimuli.

I can imagine some cases of arthritis being severe enough to warrant trying such drugs for pain, under controls and for a limited time. But these drugs do nothing to cure the disease causing the pain and may produce even more discomfort. The side effects may not show up for a while, but you cannot go on insulting living tissue again and again without causing damage. If alcohol in large or continual doses will fire up trigger points, what will powerful drugs do?

When my hip started to hurt I did the usual. I went the rounds of the doctors, and, sure enough, Indocin was prescribed

79

along with several other drugs including "muscle relaxants," which are really tranquilizers. One popular one was called Robaxin, and the pharmaceuticals house admits (in print) that its safety and effectiveness for children under the age of 12 have not been established. I wasn't under 12, but I had the distinct impression that it isn't any better for older people. The possible side effects were listed as lightheadedness, dizziness, drowsiness, nausea, rash, eye irritation, visual disturbances, nasal congestion, blurred vision, headache, and fever. All that to offset a pain in the hip.

Just reading what you might get that you haven't got now should make you most reluctant to risk your body to reckless medication. By the time I finished tabulating and looking up what all those words meant, I felt like my grandfather when he was studying to become a doctor. Day by day he contracted all the symptoms for every disease on the agenda. He eventually had to leave medical school and take up law. I shall be glad to get out of this discussion and back into myotherapy, trigger points, exercise, and improved well-being. That world is clear-cut and positive.

CASE HISTORIES OF ARTHRITICS HELPED BY MYOTHERAPY

Dolores Goodwin lives in a nursing home in New Hampshire. She lived in one or another of such places for 20 years. She was severely stricken with rheumatoid arthritis, unable even to sit upright in a chair. Her muscles, one after the other and then in bunches, went into agonizing spasm. Her hands, incredibly twisted, resembled sea anemones. They were practically useless as were her arms and legs. Her entire body was ramrod stiff and her neck riveted so that she was unable to turn her head an inch to right or left. Her legs were locked together. When I feel like complaining I think of Dolores Goodwin and the urge passes.

Two years ago we were giving a Fit for Life Workshop in Durham, New Hampshire. A Fit for Life Workshop deals with the physical problems of the aging and how to reverse the trend toward incapacitation and dependence. There is a great deal that could be done that isn't being done to bring fitness programs to older people, even the bedridden. We spend about three hours during the weekend on myotherapy. A young man who was a physiotherapist in Dolores's nursing home was very attentive.

Five weeks later I received a handwritten letter from Mrs. Goodwin telling me she didn't know how to thank me enough. The therapist, whose name was Carl, had worked on her trigger points every day and "Thank God . . ." (she counted on Him, too) she was now sitting up for the first time in 19 years. Her daughter, now 26, had wheeled her out onto the patio, and both had cried all the way. She had not seen her mother dressed and sitting up since she was seven years old.

"Look at this letter. I've written it myself! . . . And I'm able to feed myself real food." Can you imagine spending 19 years without being able to lift a spoon, sign a note, arrange a blanket, or even scratch an itch?

Two months later when we were doing a workshop at the Laconia State School for the Handicapped, we went to visit with Dolores. She knew we were coming and was sitting in front of the TV set. I introduced myself and she reached to shake my hand, but didn't look away from the set. It took me a few seconds to realize she couldn't stop looking at the TV (a fate worse than death some days). She was sitting up and could move her arms but not her head. Her neck was still in the iron collar of spasm.

We went back to her room with Carl and I worked on her neck, upper back, and chest. She could look left, right, up, and down in 15 minutes. Today, two years later, she has become a fine painter, works at her church, puts out a newsletter, and visits family and friends. She is a very happy woman, and except when in flare, free of pain.

Dolores Goodwin is out of irons, she has wheels on her chair and can get about, and is an inspiration to a lot of people. Carl continues to work with her and will be needed probably as long as she lives. She has rheumatoid, and rheumatoid is one of those diseases that attacks and then recedes. When it attacks it lays down new trigger points or fires up old ones. They of course cause spasm and pain. Relief at that time usually comes in the form of potent medication. But the body can absorb just so much of that stuff without becoming sick in other ways. If trigger points are erased from Dolores's muscles regularly, the pain is held to a minimum and so is the medication. When the disease goes into remission, she is altogether free of pain. Then too there is no need for any medication. This allows her to build herself back up to a higher level of fitness. When patients do not have such help they continue to take the medication longer than they should. We hear over and over that the object is to stop the medication as soon as possible, but we see too often that it isn't stopped soon enough.

Nursing homes are sad places at best. One of myotherapy's great contributions is keeping people out of nursing homes by helping them maintain their independence. Myotherapy can restore manual mobility to those confined to bed. It can also get many like Dolores into chairs and out into the world. It can also get many in wheelchairs back onto their feet.

Arthritis is believed to be a disease that is brought on by the body's inability to withstand and adjust to stress. One of the most dangerous forms of stress is the one we refer to as "climate," emotional stress. People with the tendency toward arthritis can be spun into an attack by loss, sorrow, hatred, loneliness, fear, anxiety, or envy as easily as they would be by an automobile accident, a mugging, or a fall from a horse.

Robert was seven when he came down with psoriatic arthritis. It was right after his father died. Psoriatic arthropatica is related to psoriasis, which is a hereditary skin disorder. The pain was excruciating and prevented the little boy from enjoying most of the fun that comes with childhood. As he grew, however, it disappeared and he looked forward to graduation and a summer of backpacking in the Wind Rivers. He never got there. The motorcycle on which he and a buddy were riding collided with a truck, and Robert spent his summer in a hospital. Nothing had been broken, but he had been severely shaken. Instead of improving as a healthy young man should have, he grew worse week by week. His pain spread from his back to all his limbs, his neck, and even his face. The arthritis had come roaring out like a bear disturbed in midwinter. When Robert finally left the hospital holding two canes in hands that barely closed over the handles, he could hardly navigate.

When Robert came to the institute he had made the rounds of hospitals, arthritis clinics, and specialists. He had tried all the available medications and given them up, preferring pain and disability to the side effects. Could we help? I didn't know. Myotherapy was still very new, and I'd never even heard of psoriatic arthritis, but we would try. I asked as always, "What would you like fixed first?"

"Well," he said without much enthusiasm, "my jaw's been clamped almost shut for over a year and I'm mighty sick of baby food." So we started with his neck and jaw, doing the work described in the previous chapter for face, neck and TMJD. In a very short while his mouth opened wide, and off he went to McDonald's for a Big Mac.

Robert came to us twice a week for five weeks. After the jaw we tackled his hands, which couldn't close efficiently and in the mornings were often so painful he wasn't able to do buttons or hold a toothbrush. The Bodo was invented for this problem. With it he could find the trigger points causing the painful spasms, and by simply putting it on the table, placing his hand or wrist on it, and bearing down, he could erase the trigger points and then the muscles would stretch.

Each day there were small but perceptible gains. One day he could sit down by bending his knees rather than straddling his straight legs and falling back onto the chair. Another day he startled his therapist by triumphantly crossing his legs. Soon he could abandon his cane. His consumption of Big Mac's was prodigious.

Success story? Yes, as far as it went, but it didn't go far enough. Because of Robert we learned we could clean out the "debris" left in muscles by arthritis attacks, but we had to work with many other sufferers who lived close by before we found that you don't get rid of arthritis, you just get rid of the pain caused by arthritis.

Robert went off into the sunset when he should have moved in down the block. When we contacted him about using his name and story in this book he was very bitter: "It didn't last."

No, it doesn't last when you have a disease that responds to stress, because stress is always present. For someone like Robert myotherapy becomes like insulin for the diabetic; it's needed on a regular basis and in doses commensurate with what happens daily. But if you can find a caring friend as many do, or grow your own therapist as Nancy Armstrong did with her daughter who treated Nancy's headaches, you need not say it didn't last, because it will.

Incidentally, in essence the story is true, but Robert is not his real name.

Eileen had a home, kids, a job, and rheumatoid. She is

both counterlady and waitress in a popular lunch place. Eileen is the major reason it's popular. Day in and day out she has a smile for everyone and a lot of Irish wit. Sometimes she has a shoulder for someone in need. Eileen had never felt well, not all well. Something always hurt. She came here for a session one day, and as I offered my hand she drew back both hers to her chest. They were swollen, knobby, and red.

"Oh, I can't shake hands. I'd like to but they hurt too much." I asked whether she had come to see me about her hands.

"No, I don't expect you to do anything for them, they've been bad for too long. It's my elbows and knees."

We began. To clear the elbows of pain we needed to start the way we do for arms, beginning in the chest, upper back, and shoulders. By the time we had worked down to the elbows, they were straight, relaxed, and free of pain. I explained that I had to be sure there was nothing lurking in the lower arm that might start the pain up again.

"Fine, but just be careful not to get too close to my hands." I was. After both arms were freed of pain, we worked on the legs, beginning in the hips as we would for backache. You can imagine her delight when half an hour later she was standing on painfree legs for the first time in years.

"Now let me look at your hands," I said as if that were the most natural thing in the world, hoping to God I would be able to work on them. "I won't hurt you any more than I already have."

She wasn't too sure about that, but she held one out. To her amazement (and mine) the swelling was already down. I started very gently, much as I do with babies. Again to our amazement, it didn't hurt one bit more than pressing on the brachioradialis at the elbow. In a matter of minutes considerable range of motion had been gained and she could flex all her fingers and her thumb—painlessly.

"Now," I said, offering my hand, "can you grip my hand?" She took hold very gently and then started to squeeze. The grip was there, the strength was there, and the warmth was there. But the pain wasn't there anymore.

That night Eileen went dancing for the first time in four years. She reminded me of the jockey who came in with a badly sprained ankle after a fall in the county-fair race. I had erased the trigger points in half an hour and suggested he rest it for twenty-four. Instead, he too went dancing.

When I asked Eileen and the jockey, too, how their legs felt after dancing, each replied, "Fine." When I asked them if they weren't worried that the pain might start up again, each replied that no, they knew I could take it away again. There is an important key there. No one should have to give up pleasures because of pain. No one should have to give up a job or freedom, independence or life because of pain. One should know how to erase pain. Then life becomes immediately less uncertain.

While a large number of people do contract arthritis, an even larger group think they have. If you do develop it, you will probably contract one of four major forms, and we have found that all four respond to myotherapy. Most of our work has been done on people who have osteoarthritis, partly because more people have it, but also because people suffering with rheumatoid tend to think in terms of medication rather than alternatives. They have been educated to think medicine.

A letter I received from a patient suffering from lupus is a case in point. Before the letter, though, a word about lupus. Lupus is identified medically as a noninfectious disease causing deterioration of the connective tissue in various parts of the body. It may attack the soft internal organs as well as bones and muscles. The cause or causes of lupus are unknown. Lupus is included in this chapter because one symptom of the disease can be arthritis in different parts of the body. It is also labeled an arthritide. An arthritide is any skin eruption of gouty or arthritic origin. Does that sound cut and dried? Even my grandfather could read that without developing a symptom, but read what Julia, a lupus sufferer, has to say about a disease that can ravage utterly. A disease that can cause so much pain that the sufferer will often settle for anything that relieves the pain.

> Actually I feel myself in a sort of limbo. The medical fraternity is responsible for a great deal of my stress since I get nothing from them but frustration and more medication. However, now that they have hooked me, if I try to phase down by as little as 1 mg. of prednisone I'm up the wall. And what frightens me is that I read that if I permit the inflammation to continue, this in turn will lead to deformity and lack of function,

85

which I can ill afford. It is my right hand that is most seriously affected, and I'd become a basket case if I couldn't do for myself.

Well, my hair looks like gray-black barbed wire. Can't do anything with it. I wash and set it and in an hour it's right back to wire. The doctor tells me it's what is known as "lupus hair." Isn't that a way to set a fella up!? And I can't wear short-sleeved anything for fear they will think I got this way at Buchenwald.

Fat face, rotten hair, hands that look like they belong on a ninety-year-old, fat deposits on my tummy, bloodshot eyes and withered arms. I know it sounds like I have an overdeveloped ego, but what female doesn't want to look her best?! These things make me look like a careless, sloppy old biddy—and I've always tried to make the very best of what I was given to start with.

I've reached the point where the AMA has nothing to offer me except trade-offs, trade one ailment for something worse. There are jillions of books on arthritis, and I've started to read some of them. They all end up the same way, a great many words and platitudes, really nothing new, nothing I haven't already heard. The vitamin bit and various approaches to holistic are (a) long term for vitamin therapy and preventive rather than corrective, and (b) holistic is faith healer type and I have no faith.

What I believe I am suffering from at this point is depression and searching for a way of life—in view of the fact that everything that mattered has been taken away. In addition to the present problems, for a long time I've been afflicted with painful feet. Only by wearing very comfortable, cushiony, cheepie shoes am I able to walk without a great deal of misery. This, plus lupus rules out tennis, which was the one sport I enjoyed. The sun is now my enemy and heretofore the sun always made me look better and feel better because I looked better. Now one glance at the mirror and my day is finished.

I just can't get myself to socialize and have long ago cut myself off from any possible activity, so it's to work and back. Now I start to worry about how long I'll be able to manage that. I wonder too, how long one can live in a total vacuum?

This is a very capable businesswoman whose children are grown and flown. She was widowed a couple of years ago, but continues to run her very successful manufacturing plant. She was always smartly dressed, beautifully groomed, and slim. In today's vernacular, she was very "with it."

I knew myotherapy could help, and I wrote her to come. She did and I was more shocked by her "new" appearance than I cared to admit even to myself. All the things she described were all too visible, but it was her gait that shook me the most. She stumped along on totally "frozen" feet. There was no motion at all in the feet, and the big toes were pulled toward the middle of each foot with large bunions destroying their forward line. She had to be helped down the four steps leading to my living room.

I asked my usual question when I know just everything hurts: "What shall I fix first?" By that I imply that I can, and I also find out where hopes lie. Remember, Eileen didn't think I could help her hands. I was to find out that Julia didn't have any hope for her feet. They had been painful even before she had developed lupus.

"Well, my arms are just terrible. I guess that's where we should start."

She got onto the table very slowly and carefully and lay face down so I could work on her upper back (where work on arms should begin). I found her back, as I had known I would, a mass of trigger points. I erased the trigger points and then did the same for her arms, which were equally riddled.

"Now, would you turn over please?" I said. In response, she propped herself up on one arm as any painfree person would do in preparation for turning. Her mouth dropped open in surprise.

"My God! I haven't done that in I can't remember how long. Look, I'm actually leaning on my arm. And it doesn't hurt!"

It took about an hour to clear most of her muscles of the trigger points and to stretch out the hitherto spasmed muscles. Then I looked at her feet.

"You have a long second toe," I told her. "Dr. Travell calls what you have a 'classic Greek foot' because all the Greek statues have them. It's also called 'Morton's Toe.' It's a lousy foot."

She said that she knew there had to be something wrong with her feet. They were terribly painful, but what had that to do with the length of her second toe? Just about everything, I

87

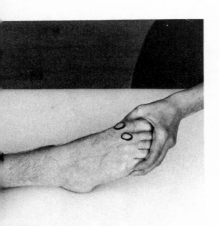

told her, and that, happily, the treatment after myotherapy costs roughly a dollar and ten cents.

THE CLASSIC GREEK FOOT

In the "classic Greek foot" the second metatarsal is longer than the first. Usually, as it is in the Greek statuary, the toe is also longer, but the joint can be longer even when the second toe is the same length as or shorter than the big toe. To be sure that your second-toe joint is not producing a hidden Greek foot, bend all your toes downward and check the metatarsals. If the second metatarsal appears to be farther forward than the joint in the big toe, you have it. Now let's examine what it does and what it has to do with arthritis (and sports and dance and gout, and walking and jogging, and balance—and pain).

A "good" foot provides the solid base of a tripod. Your weight comes down on your heel with each step, and as the weight is transferred forward, it lands on the ball of the foot just back of the big toe and also on the outside edge of the metatarsal arch. Such a foot can take many such steps without tiring. A "good" foot is a very handy thing to have.

Now what of the classic Greek foot? With that foot the weight does not shift forward onto two points, but onto a single point in the metatarsal arch just under the second metatarsal, which is in the middle of the front of the foot. There are several signs that announce this problem, and two of the first are poor balance and "growing pains." As the child grows and we lock his or her feet into boxes called shoes, the problem is exacerbated, and the foot, grabbing for stability, develops a hard callous on the outside of the big toe.

Instead of resting on a tripod, the foot with the long second toe stands on a knife edge, teetering with each step. The effort to maintain balance lays trigger points in the tibialis anterior (see Plate 7 or 9 in Appendix 1). The ankle, overstressed and never quite stable, is easily sprained. Since the ankle joint is unstable, the knee joint is also, and its efforts to achieve stability lay down trigger points in the quadriceps, the huge muscles of the thigh. That isn't the end of it either. The next joint above is the hip joint, which also has to work too hard to hold the body correctly on so shaky a base. That, of course, can provide pain anywhere, as various muscle groups go into spasm.

Meanwhile, as the years pass, a callus forms in the middle of the metatarsal arch and the diagnosis is fallen arches. One way to handle that problem is to stick a pad right on top of the callus, which effectively increases the instability. Many people have their calluses sliced off periodically, which isn't quite as bad, but does nothing for the *cause* of the condition, so of course, it returns.

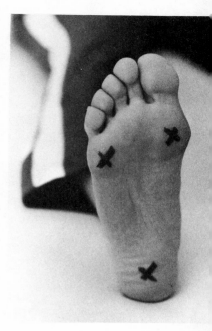

Fairly early on the big toe begins to turn toward the other four and this ultimately becomes a bunion. The second toe, grabbing all the while, also develops a callus and often a condition known as hammertoe. Whenever there is constant strain, there is repeated trauma, and trauma lays the groundwork for arthritis. Julia's feet were perfect examples of every one of these unpleasant symptoms. Had an X-ray been taken, the pictures would almost assuredly have shown arthritis, but she didn't even need an X-ray; she had "arthritis," right? And arthritis ruins feet, doesn't it? The family doctor had told her that she had arthritis, the rheumatologist had told her she had arthritis, even she agreed she had arthritis. But that wasn't the cause of the foot pain. Trigger points in the muscles of the feet and legs were the cause of the foot pain.

Half an hour later we had cleaned out most of the spasm and then came the dollar and ten cent "cure." We got out a pair of those Dr. Scholl's innersoles, size seven, to fit her shoes. Then we cut a circle about the size of a quarter from one-eighth-inch sponge rubber with stickum on one side. We stuck that to the innersole at the spot where the ball of the foot should strike as the weight moves forward. To that circle we glued a second one about the size of a nickel. The main thing is to see that the circles do not encroach on the area of the second metatarsal. One wants the weight *off* the spot where the callus is.

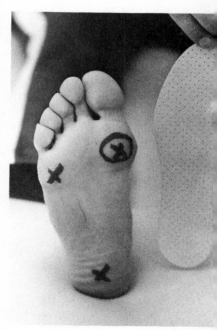

So many minor miracles had already befallen Julia, her arms were free of pain, her neck had full range, her color was vastly improved, and the pain was gone not only from her body, but from her face as well. We got her back into her clothes and the doctored shoes. As she faced her reflection in a full-length mirror, I said, "All right. Now walk." And walk she did, but she seemed hardly to touch the floor.

89

The man who had brought her up to see us was an old and dear friend. He had been greatly troubled by her condition and appearance. He and several of my students were waiting for her in the living room. I turned on the radio, which is always tuned to our music station. Everyone looked toward the stairs and the shoji screen that afforded her a stage entrance. Gone was the stumbling gait, the tightly held torso, and the bent shoulders. She came across the floor and skipped down the four steps she had been helped up only two hours before. She whirled along the full 35-foot length of the room coming to a most theatrical stop with a "bump"! Now no woman does a "bump" in public unless she is perfectly sure of herself. Does that sound like the woman who wrote the letter?

Here is a second letter, in part, that came a week later.

I came not as a doubting Thomas, but with reservations. Having been to several specialists, none of whom had any suggestions other than prednisone while admitting it does nothing to stem the disease, but merely controls the pain. With lupus the pain can be excruciating, so even that would have been a welcome relief were it not for the dreadful side effects which are cumulative.

And now, myotherapy, the first remedy I've encountered that made sense. Here we are repairing the damage, helping the body help itself. It was a revelation to note the difference in sensation between pressure in the non-affected areas and pressure where obviously there was spasm. Though there was a certain amount of pain, the relief after the therapy went beyond just that and was an overall exhilaration of the whole body. There had been no strength in my upper arms to support my torso if I wanted to raise up on my elbow. Shortly after you started your work I was up on my elbow without realizing it and my shoulders were free of pain, and functioning.

I guess the reaction to the handling of my feet was the most startling. I wasn't even going to mention that my feet had been my greatest problem for years, and I was contemplating listening to information about some supposed remedies through surgery—out of sheer desperation.

Now of course I'm not naive enough to expect that such results after only one session could correct the ills accumulated over years, but I do believe that periodic application of myotherapy administered either by myself or someone trained to do it could eventually replace the drug therapy and permit my body to help repair itself.

Like many others whose disease may go into remission but won't ever be cured, Julia will be carried on "maintenance" at the institute. She will be able to keep the pain under control with myotherapy and will need medication only when the disease is in flare. But that isn't all. Though her disease can't be cured, her depression has been. As evidenced in her second letter, Julia now has hope. Moreover, because her body can move without giving her pain, she will be able to exercise. The exercise will restore her once-strong muscles and take the fat from her abdomen. In time, when she is off the medication, the "moon face" will once again have its high cheekbones and firm lines. Her hair will regain its healthy texture, and, while tennis may not be for her anymore, she will socialize again.

WHAT MODERN MEDICINE HAS IN ITS LITTLE BLACK BAG FOR ARTHRITICS

Complete bed rest is rarely proposed, thank goodness! There is too much danger of muscle and joint atrophy. If hips or knees are affected it will probably be recommended that long walks and stair climbing be avoided. This is not much of a denial to people who don't like walking anyway and never climbed a mountain. For walkers and climbers, it is.

The addition of a cane or a change to "orthopedic" shoes might not bother a man, but as you saw in Julia's letter, considerable damage can be done to a woman's psyche. Most of the suggestions are for palliatives, which neither cure disease nor erase pain.

Physical therapy may be offered, but it would be well to find out what your doctor means by physical therapy for you, and what the physical therapist means. A friend of mine was subjected to lifting weights after hip surgery. That particular exercise effectively sent her muscles into spasm, which tore the new hip joint apart, adding painful years, another operation, and more painful years after that. Many of the people who come to the institute for myotherapy have had physiotherapy for months

91

without positive results. Most of the methods used are palliative: heat, electrical stimulation, counterirritants, whirlpool baths, and hot paraffin. None gets at the real cause. Painful hands soaked in hot whirling water or paraffin may feel eased for the moment, but the cause of the pain, trigger points in the upper arms, will be back on the job by the following day, if not before.

Diathermy has lost its popularity, but if the PT department still has one of the machines, it may be used anyway. The patient is paying for something and he'd better get something whether it works or not. There is no proof that elevating the temperatures deep within the tissues with high frequency current, ultrasonic waves, or microwave radiation does anything at all. It is my feeling that radiation of any kind is cumulative, and one is never sure when "enough" is really "too much." Only the years can tell us that, and then it will be too late to correct.

Exercise will also be offered, but exercise is often mishandled. To start with, exercise applied to muscles in spasm is barbaric. The pain is excruciating, and the exercise will only worsen the spasm anyway. Before any exercise, even gentle passive stretch, get the trigger points causing the spasm to stop firing. Only then will painless, and therefore productive, exercise be possible.

And then, what exercise is right? Doctors are deficient when it comes to knowledge of exercise. Medical schools in America do not provide courses on exercise, the colleges do not provide it, the high schools do not provide it nor do the lower schools. Some physicians suggest isometric exercise, but except for tightening the abdominals and buttocks in a pelvic tilt, I think it's harmful. It limits the supply of blood to the muscles and works against stretch, which hurt muscles badly need.

What is needed are exercises that put the body through the full range of motion painlessly, exercises that develop sufficient strength to withstand the stresses we impose on our muscles. Sometimes in order to increase the range of motion a patient will be put into traction. Unfortunately, traction lays down its own trigger points and rarely relieves pain caused by spasm.

Operations for arthritis have made an enormous difference in the lives of millions, and I am one of them. Since I have talked a lot about my two total hip replacements on TV I have built up quite a correspondence with "hippies." They are people who are going to have a hip replaced, should have one replaced, or have had one replaced. Many are young, and their doctors are reluctant to do the job. Their reasoning is that, since the best way to make a hip functional again is to destroy what is left and replace the joint with metal and plastic, the young body may outlast the hip. Because they want the replacement to outlast the patient, they prefer to wait until the patient is so old that it most likely will. To my mind this is medical, not sensible, thinking. I ran into that thinking with my first hip when I was 58.

Crippling is bad at any age, but it seems to me it would be better to have it happen later than earlier. I figured that at 58 I wanted to be as active as possible (and that's very active), and Dr. Travell was right in there with me. "Have it done and run. If it breaks down get that one replaced. By the time it happens, who knows, they may have discovered something even better."

Young people who are courting, building careers, and raising families, need legs free from pain. The doctor who is withholding an operation from a 20- to 40-year-old knows nothing of constant pain, crutches, and interference with sex drive. If the patient is on one of the potent drugs we have discussed in this chapter, it may well result in the total loss of sex drive, among other problems.

There are other surgical interventions in use—all those described here being for the treatment of osteoarthritis. Surgery to treat rheumatoid is discussed later.

Debridement is the removal of all damaged and excess tissue from the joint.

Athrodesis is the fusing of a joint to give it stability.

Arthroplasty is the insertion of a piece of plastic or metal between the working surfaces of a damaged joint to make motion painless. Before the coming of the Charnley Total Hip Replacement in the sixties and seventies (mine in the seventies was still "experimental"), the "cup arthroplasty" was the only way to fix a hip. Arthur Godfrey had one of those, and through him I learned it had definite limitations. About 30 percent of them didn't work at all, and it took months of painful exercise to rehabilitate patients in whom it did work.

Since those days many improvements have been made, and my newest hip replacement is the American Harris Total Hip Replacement. So now there is an English Charnley teamed with the American Harris in the same pelvis, and I must say they work well together.

In one year 80,000 artificial hips were used to replace joints destroyed by arthritis and other diseases. There is a one percent failure due to infection. The overall ten-year failure rate is 5 percent. Thousands of knee replacements have been done. Elbow and shoulder replacements are rarer, but several thousand knuckles are replaced every year.

Surgery for rheumatoid arthritis is a different kettle of fish altogether. It is done to relieve pain and correct deformity. The woman who came to the institute to see if anything could be done for her legs and feet, the one who soon walked down the hill and back, was terribly deformed. Her tortured, contracted shoulders were half as wide as mine, and on each elbow was a lump about the size of half an orange. In surgery, such a growth could be removed. Surgery could have restored her joint function to a degree, but it is pain, not loss of function, that is the major indication for surgery in rheumatoid. Pain is a great decider. When I was told in 1966 that my arthritic hip would eventually have to be replaced I asked, "How soon?" The answer was terse and direct, "Pain will dictate." It sure did!

In surgery for rheumatoid, greater mobility is welcomed gladly if it comes, but it is not really expected. The rehabilitation is long and arduous, but that may change with the use of myotherapy to erase the pain and facilitate exercise. The physiotherapy in use today is still palliative, which is half an answer at best.

I believe that when arthritis has destroyed a joint, the best course is to replace it, and without delay. The long, usually hopeless struggle to put off the operation is terribly costly in pain, fatigue, and additional damage to other joints that must do the work of two. I receive a lot of mail, however, from people in their early sixties. They need the operation, all right, and have opted for it, but can't afford it. So they are waiting until their medical bills will be taken over by Medicare. Such a situation puts them into a miserable holding pattern of pain, potential drug addiction, and subjugation to the poisonous side effects of powerful medication.

Their best bet is myotherapy—and myotherapy done on a regular basis since the disease will continually rekindle any extinguished trigger points—then, "into the pool," so to speak. Whirlpool baths and baths in hot tubs, which are merely palliative, have only water in common with what I'm about to suggest.

94

Photo credit: Clemens Kalischer

The body must move to be healthy. The body in pain cannot move against gravity without increasing pain, but in water the body is weightless. When exercise is done in water, the joints and muscles can be put through great range of motion. The major problem is temperature. Muscles either in spasm or with the tendency to spasm should be kept out of cold water. The temperature of the pool water at Y's and hotels is usually in the vicinity of 80°, which isn't bad. If your Y has a Baby-Swim-and-Gym program, which usually takes place first thing in the morning, the water will be 85° or over. That's much better. Use the exercises in the Aqua-Ex section in Chapter 9, and if you can, tape some music you like to exercise to. You don't need much room for your workout. My own pool is 5 feet by 7 feet by 4½ feet.

If you are flush (or have a carpenter friend) consider one of those big wooden hot tubs so popular in California. There is also a cheaper way to get the benefit of a tub. Buy a small backyard pool and put it in the basement. It would be lovely to have a circulating hot water heater, but if you can't swing it, just let a foot or so of water out of the pool night and morning and add a foot of very hot water from the tap. Use it at least twice a day. Aqua-Ex won't cure the diseased joint, but it can keep your body supple and strong and your circulation good. Then should you find yourself being pushed along the hall to the operating room, you will know you did your part. You'll be as fit as you can be.

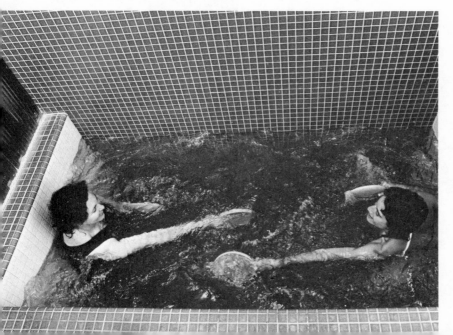

7. Common Pains and What to Do About Them

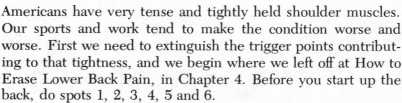

Most people have some pain. Because of poor musculature and worse nutrition, our bodies have amassed hordes of trigger points from innumerable minor strains.

Backaches were rare for the man who mowed the lawn with a hand mower, trimmed the walks on his hands and knees, and shoveled coal into the hopper, took out the ashes in a bucket, and worked six days a week. So were heart attacks. And so was chronic pain elsewhere in his body.

But we have chronic pain now, and it's at epidemic proportions. How shall we handle it? Let's get rid of it. Here's how.

SHOULDER-PAIN SYNDROME

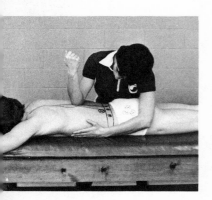

Americans have very tense and tightly held shoulder muscles. Our sports and work tend to make the condition worse and worse. First we need to extinguish the trigger points contributing to that tightness, and we begin where we left off at How to Erase Lower Back Pain, in Chapter 4. Before you start up the back, do spots 1, 2, 3, 4, 5 and 6.

Referring to Plate 5 in Appendix 1, we proceed up the back at one-inch intervals along the dotted lines shown above spots 7 and 8. Don't forget to do both sides of the back even if there's no pain at all, and especially if there is pain on only one side. Use the elbow until you reach the neck and are ready to tackle the scapula (shoulder blade).

The latissimus dorsi is another important muscle, if only for its size: There is an enormous amount of acreage in which trigger points can hide. Grid E on Plate 5 and drawn here on Rick's back will locate the latissimus dorsi for you. The work should be done systematically. Use the squares in the grid to keep track of where your elbow has been, and try to be thorough.

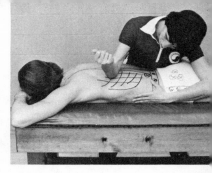

In the next technique, erasing trigger points along the top of the shoulder, if a small myotherapist is working on a big subject, additional leverage may be needed, especially when the subject is a top athlete. The elbow is placed in position at the top of the shoulder, and then pull exerted on the subject's arm to augment the push. Hold for the usual seven seconds and move outward on spots 16, 15, and 14, shown on Plate 5. Do both sides.

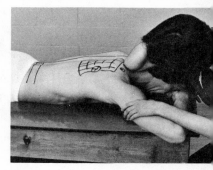

Just below the crest of the shoulder, over which is draped the trapezius, we have grid D, the upper back, also shown in Plate 5. Treat it as you did the latissimus dorsi, hunting for trigger points in every square. Somewhere a little outside of center, over the scapula (shoulder blade), you will find a trigger point of the "horror" class. That is because that spot is another crossroads similar to the one in the back of the head. The "horror" is spot 13 on Plate 5. In that spot edges of the deltoid, trapezius, infraspinatus, teres minor, teres major, and latissimus dorsi are all crossing. Press straight down, but take it easy in the first session.

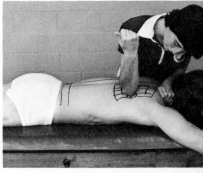

Scapula (Shoulder Blade)

Lots of unpleasantness to do with shoulder pain lurks *under* the scapula. Have the subject put his or her lower arm— the one on the side where you are working—across the back at the waist. This will have the effect of opening up the underside of the scapula so you can slide searching fingers in underneath to find tender spots.

The teres major figures in almost all sports, almost all manual labor, almost all close work, and all aborted accidents when the car did not go off the road because the driver was able to drag it out of the ditch by sheer "strength." The teres, spot 12 on Plate 5, very often has one or two excitable trigger points. They are best found by using your fingers. Stand on the opposite

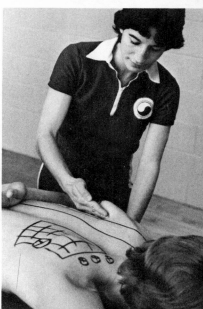

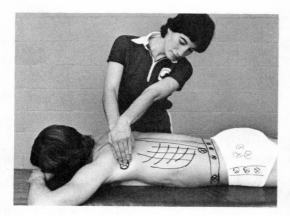
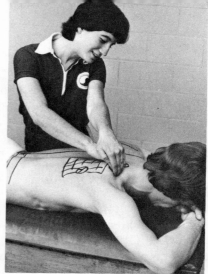

side from the work area, and for greater strength and control, cover the working fingers with those of the other hand.

Another place where the two-handed technique is helpful is at the top of the trapezius in spot 25, shown on Plate 6. Use the pulling-down action with as much force as possible when you are dealing with athletes. For lesser physical specimens, less strength is necessary.

At this stage as always, once the trigger point erasure is completed, it must be followed by stretching exercises, a wide variety of which the shoulders require.

THE THREAD-NEEDLE STRETCH

The subject kneels on all fours and reaches through with the right hand into the space between the left arm and thigh. Then the arm is withdrawn and flung straight up as the eyes follow the hand. Do four to a side. This exercise stretches the chest and back and improves range of motion in the shoulders. Don't forget, to relieve shoulder pain you will also have to work on the chest and the neck, but most especially on the arms.

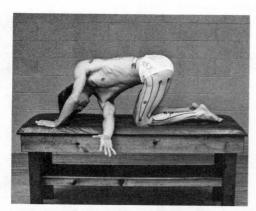
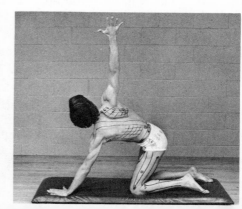

SHRUG SERIES

These are the best exercises we have for tense and painful shoulders and should always be done after working on the shoulders, upper back, chest, neck, and arms. Do them often throughout the day.

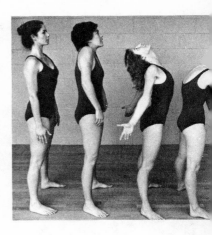

1. Round the back by dropping the head forward. At the same time twist the arms inward and bring the backs of the arms as close together as possible in front of the body.
2. Stretch both arms back with thumbs leading, to stretch the chest. Tip the head back.
3. Pull the shoulders up to the ears as if trying to cover them.
4. Press the shoulders down *hard* to make a long neck.

Do the "shrug series" four times after myotherapy, but don't stop there. Tension builds up throughout the day. Don't wait until you feel a burning thread of pain in one shoulder to exercise the tension away. That's too late. Tie it in with your daily tasks. Do the series before you leave your desk. If you are working in the house, then between bed-making and dusting and again before starting lunch. You will also need the shoulder-rotation exercises on page 122.

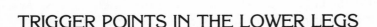

TRIGGER POINTS IN THE LOWER LEGS

Legs have a great deal to do with backache, and the heating pad of today is just about as helpful as the mustard plaster was way back when. Getting a special seat for your car and wearing a corset are equally unsuccessful if you don't rid yourself of the cause of the pain—the trigger points.

Most people have trigger points in their lower legs. All the women I have checked who wore high heels most of the time had them. All the men who were athletes had them, and only one woman athlete did not. She had no trigger points anywhere although a fine skier and gymnast. (She did develop them in her shoulders when she went to work for city hall and found her muscles, nerves, and humor tightly constricted by reams of red tape!)

People who have a long second toe have trigger points in the legs, as do dancers. Anyone who has leg or foot spasms, and anyone who has sprained any part of the leg, broken a toe, or

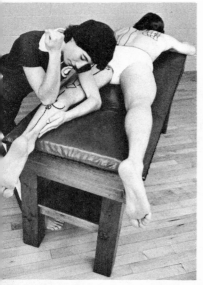

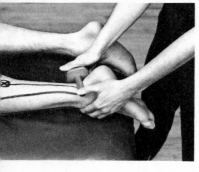

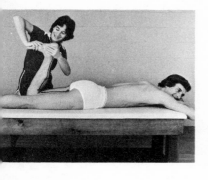

ever had hip problems will be found to have them. Also, people with cerebral palsy or multiple sclerosis, or arthritis that has affected the legs. Anyone who overuses the legs—cabbies, truckers, organists, and dentists—will have them. Does that leave anyone? The safest route is just to figure you have them and erase them or at least get them under control. Otherwise, you can expect to be joining that vast army of older people taking medication for night cramps.

Turn to Plate 8 in Appendix 1, the lower leg. You will see that the gastrocnemius (the calf muscle) has two heads. It is the nesting place of one of the two worst trigger points in the lower leg, so that's where the work begins.

Have your subject lie prone. Place your elbow in the center of the gastrocnemius at spot 45, just below the bulge.

If the instep is tight, avoid straining it by putting a pillow or rolled towel under the ankle. If the subject is elderly it is best to rest the entire leg on a pillow plus the rolled towel under the ankle. Elderly legs are often thin and, until you clear them, replete with spasm.

Once you have erased spot 45, go down the leg at one-inch intervals on the center line shown on plate 8. At the point where the muscles run into the Achilles tendon, the thick cord down near the ankle, you will find using a Bodo helpful. Just lay it across the top of the cord, and, while holding it in position with one hand, you press down with the thumb of the other.

LOWER-LEG STRETCH

When you have worked down to the heel, the muscles will need stretching. Bend the knee and at the same time press down on the front part of the foot. Release and then stretch again. Do the stretch three times.

The Lower Leg Continued

There are three lines running the entire length of the back of the leg. One is directly in the center. You have just run down part of that line. Starting in the gastrocs at spot 46, work your way up to the popliteal, the back of the knee. Repeat the same lower-leg stretch three more times.

If you were to cut across the top of the lower leg so that the big gastrocnemius muscle, the one you have been working on, could be peeled back, you would find another long muscle under it, also running down to the Achilles tendon. The name of this lovely is the soleus. Actually, it is indeed a lovely muscle and contributes to the dancer's gracefully pointed toe. The only trouble with it is that it is unconsciously tightened when anyone in a sitting position concentrates.

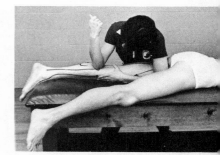

To erase trigger points along it, we start at the top of the inner aspect of the back of the leg, at spot 47 as shown on Plate 8. Go down the line that passes through it, at one-inch intervals, right into the heel. The Bodo will be helpful around the ankle. Do the same lower-leg stretch exercise but with the foot turned out.

The third line for the back of the lower leg, the one toward the outside, starts at spot 47A. This is not usually very painful, but we "search" it anyway, just on the off chance that a one-time sprain or strain left a little something in there. Travel down that line at one-inch intervals into the heel. Follow with the stretch exercise but this time with the foot turned in.

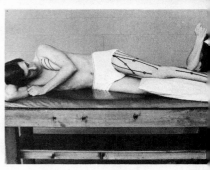

To avoid laying down any new trigger points there, try to remember that the soleus, whose real job is to flex your ankle, hears you worry. Learn to relax your legs when you work. If the job is really tough, get one of those little parking-meter gadgets that you can set for an hour, or better yet, a half hour. A kitchen timer or a clock will also do. If your friends ask you what the gadget is for, tell them you do two or three exercises every time it goes off and by so doing, keep the muscles relaxed and free from pain. The best exercise for tightness in the lower leg is the half knee bend. Keep your heels on the floor and pelvis tucked under and do many.

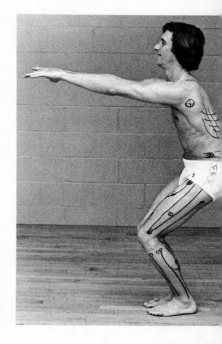

TRIGGER POINTS IN THE UPPER LEGS

There's a dilly of a trigger point here, too, and it is at spot 36 shown on Plate 8. It can be reached from the near side. The muscles you will be leaning on are the adductor magnus, which adducts and extends the thigh, and the semitendinosus, which flexes the leg and extends the thigh. Most people have a bad trigger point in there, and all horse riders we have worked with have them. That would be logical, as the necessity of keeping

101

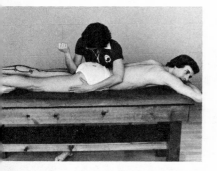

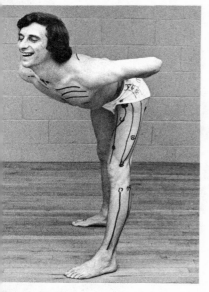

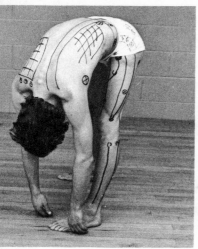

the knees "on," or against the horse's flanks, is constant. If the horse should shy or stumble, the adductors could be strained. Not if, but when, a woman has a baby she will hear from this one, and also any she has been so foolish as to overlook in the gluteals, which connect nearby.

Start at spot 36 and proceed down the leg at one-inch intervals. If spot 36 reacts, you may be sure that there will be others in that line.

FLEXIBILITY BOUNCES TO THE SIDE

Stand with the feet wide apart and clasp hands behind your back. Keeping the knees straight and the head up, turn your upper body to the left. Do eight easy bounces in this direction. Straighten up and then do the same exercise to the other side, even if you have not detriggered that side. You will in a minute.

Drop the upper body over the left leg and repeat the eight bounces. Then to the other side. Those two exercises make up a set. Do one set each time a line in the upper leg is worked over. A line runs from the top of the thigh down to the popliteal in the back of the knee.

The Upper Leg, Part II

Spot 37, which starts the line between the muscles that flex the leg and extend the thigh, can be rough. They are the biceps femoris and the vastus lateralis. The latter is notorious as a nest of trouble for basketball and tennis players and anyone else who must change direction speedily while running. Dancers, runners, and football players are also wont to overwork these muscles. Start at the top and work down to the popliteal at one-inch intervals.

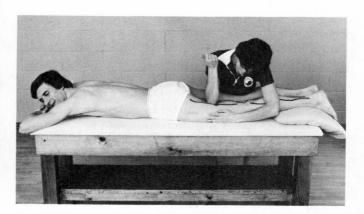

FLEXIBILITY BOUNCES TO THE SIDE WITH SHOULDER DROP

The exercise for stretching the muscles you have just cleared is similar to the stretch just used for the inside of the leg, with one important difference. Start in the spread-leg position, hands behind your back and your head up as before. But now, drop your left shoulder. You will find that your right foot may tend to roll over onto its outer edge. Do your eight bounces to the right and then to the left for one set.

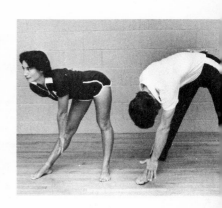

Follow these with eight bounces to the right, but this time, drop the entire upper body and left arm. Keep the right arm across the back at the waist. Do eight of these to the left as well.

The Upper Leg, Part III

The third line on the back of the upper leg starts at spot 38 and runs right down the middle, ending at the popliteal. It hits the edges of the biceps femoris, semitendinosus, and semimembranosus.

FLEXIBILITY BOUNCES STRAIGHT ON

Follow your trigger point work with stretching. Stand with feet apart and knees straight. Clasp your hands behind your back. Keeping your head up, bounce the upper part of your body downward in eight easy bounces. Now drop the upper body straight down, letting gravity do the pulling. Those two parts make up a set. Do three sets often throughout the day.

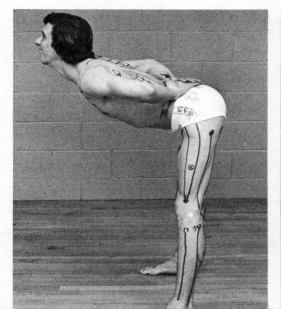
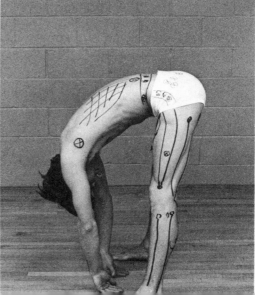

The back of the leg should now be clear, but be sure to do both legs. In some way, incomprehensible at this time, one leg seems to be able to influence the other so that undone work will undo what has been done.

RELIEF OF MENSTRUAL CRAMPS AND PAIN IN THE GROIN

Very few people think of the groin when they have a backache. After all, a groin is in front. The fact is, however, trouble in that area can readily refer pain to the back, just as a backache can affect the groin. The back contributes to menstrual cramps and can even produce a pain remarkably like gall bladder pain.

One of my new students heard me say I had found that trigger points caused menstrual cramps and that they could be erased permanently. That was spectacular news to her. "Would you please try?" she asked, because she was in a lot of pain, as are many girls and women, every month of their young and middle years. Of course I would. I did the following.

Look at spot 27 on Plate 6 in Appendix 1, the iliopsoas. You are still technically working in the leg, but very close to the pelvis rim, which supports the torso. Place your elbow or fingers on the spot designated by spot 27; it takes in the edges of the sartorius and the psoas. The sartorius is the longest muscle you have, and it flexes the thigh and leg. The psoas flexes the trunk and flexes and rotates the thigh. It attaches to the second and third lumbar vertebrae, the very best place for menstrual backache. It is sometimes difficult to find the exact spot where the trigger point is hiding. Press down and then move very slowly and carefully first in one direction and then the other. When you find the right spot, the subject will let you know! Do first one side and then the other.

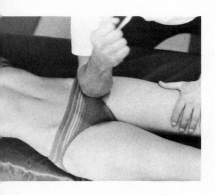

GROIN STRETCH
After searching for trigger points in this area, have your subject move to the far side of the table and hang her leg over the edge. Support the body on the table by moving in close and placing one hand on the hip bone and the other on the hanging thigh. Press down with both hands and hold for about three seconds.

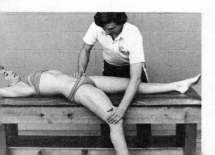

Release and repeat the stretch for another three seconds. The stretch should be done to both sides.

Next we move on to the pubic arch, spot 28 on Plate 6. Look again at Plate 1, the skeleton, and you will see that the pubic bones are not really all of a piece. They are joined together by ligaments. The joining point is the most sensitive point on the pubic arch. Place your elbow or fingers carefully and make sure you are dead center and on the bone. Don't slip off in either direction. Press down carefully and hold. The pressure should be light at first. The subject will tell you in no uncertain terms how much to use. Move outward about an inch for spot 29, also shown on Plate 6, and repeat the pressure. Do both sides. When you have finished with spots 28 and 29, repeat the groin stretch to both sides.

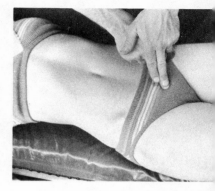

You learned the wraparound earlier, when you did it on the orbicularis oculi, the muscle around the eye. Apply that technique now to the pubic arch. Use all four fingers of both hands and reach into the pelvis bowl by starting on the rim of the arch. Wrap around over the rim and then pull the muscle back against it. Hold the required seven seconds as usual, and then move both hands as a unit one inch to the left and repeat. Do the same to the right and follow with the groin stretch once more to each side.

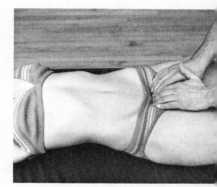

By this time any menstrual cramps should be gone, but remember that muscles have at least two attachments. If we neglect any of them, next day or next month the cramps will be back. The upper reaches of the abdominals attach to the ribs. If there are trigger points there, they will light up the ones you have just extinguished. You can use either the wraparound technique or your thumbs. Unless your subject is elderly, don't be afraid to go in under the ribs. In the case of an elderly subject, be very gentle. Ribs are sometimes brittle. Older people very often have sharp and sudden pains in the side (stitches) like the ones you get from running. This technique works wonders for both kinds of pain. Do both sides.

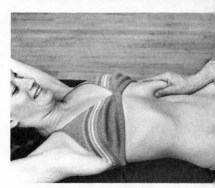

The abdominals have several layers, and just anywhere in those layers there could be trigger points. Think of the abdominals covered with the same type of grid seen on Rick's back for the latissimus dorsi (see under Shoulder Pain Syndrome in this chapter) and make a thorough search using fingers.

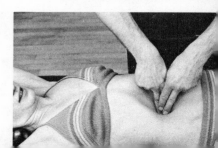

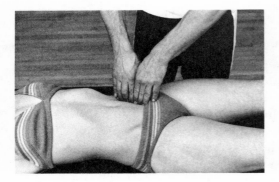

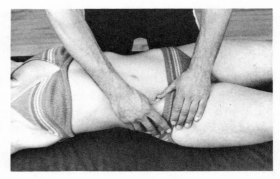

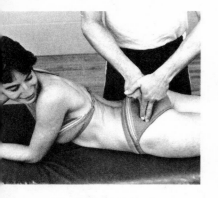

The rim of the pelvis can be searched with fingers if you work on the near side and thumbs if you are crossing over. If you check with Plate 19, showing the pelvis floor, you know full well how many muscles attach in that area.

By this time you should be pretty clear in front and will probably never suffer a stitch in your side again from running. However, to be safe from menstrual cramps, you have three more areas to search.

The gluteals, at fault so often when there is pain, play a part in menstrual cramps as well. Be very thorough, using either fingers or elbow to search for trigger points. Also pay close attention to spot 11 just above the belt (see Plate 5). Do both sides.

Lastly, work on the adductor magnus at the top of the thigh, spot 36, shown on Plate 8.

While you have just completed the series that gets rid of menstrual cramps you have also completed the series to be used prenatally (see Chapter 8 on pregnancy). Nobody should go into the delivery room without first having been detriggered. The last month before D-Day should be used for trigger point work and lots of stretch exercise.

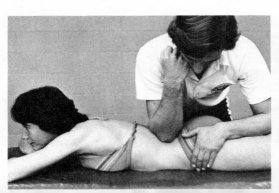

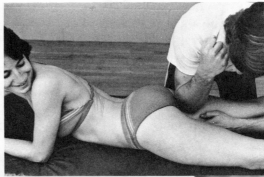

HELP FOR PAINFUL KNEES

Because the pain is in the knee most people who have painful knees are sure the trouble is in the knee. Sometimes it is. We think that more often it isn't, but rather in the muscles surrounding the knee. These muscles in spasm for whatever reason, injury or disease, pull on the joint and the joint registers pain. It also often displays swelling, clicking, rustling, and "locking." Many knees are said to "go out." Let's take a look at the map for the inside view of the leg, Plate 10 in Appendix 1.

Spot 33, on the vastus medialis, is very close to the point where that muscle and the sartorius cross. It weighs in as Horror No. 3, along with splenius capitis (spot 66 in the back of the head) and infraspinatus (spot 13 in the upper back). They are captains of two other teams of muscles causing exquisite pain.

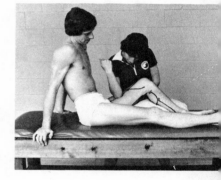

Place the bent leg on its side with a pillow under the knee. Press *gently at first* on spot 33. There is *always* a trigger point there; you registered your first one when someone gave your thigh a "horse bite" when you were about ten.

Work your way at one-inch intervals along the line starting at spot 33 right up into the groin. Follow that by working down along the same line into the knee.

It is important to remember that the inside has its opposite, the outside. Spot 39 (see Plate 9, the outside view of the leg) will be the most painful spot on the outside of the upper leg, and also the most important. That seems to be a rule of thumb. If a muscle does important work, it seems to do a lot of it. If it is overworked, and never receives the recompense due a good worker in the form of massage, myotherapy, and either exercise or counteracting exercise, then it becomes the most painful spot of all.

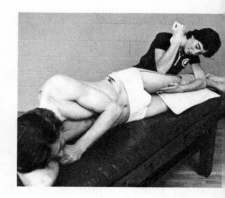

With a pillow between the subject's knees, place your elbow at spot 39 as shown. Work up to the top of the leg, pressing at one-inch intervals. Then, beginning one inch below spot 39, press at the same intervals down to the knee. (If you were using the stripe of warm-up pants as your guide, you would be right on the mark.)

Spot 35 (see Plate 7) is where work on the center of the front of the leg begins. Press at one-inch intervals, moving straight up the middle of the rectus femoris and crossing over the sartorius, right up into the groin. All sorts of surprises may

107

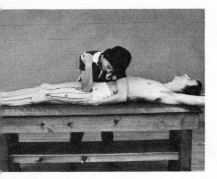

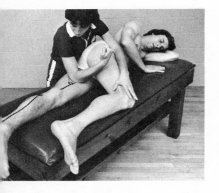

lurk along your way, none of them pleasant, but all very important to the person wanting painfree knees at whatever age.

Begin next at spot 34 (also on Plate 7), on the lateral side of the knee, and work right up to the attachment of the sartorius, again at one-inch intervals. The line moves along the tensor fascae, and a witch's coven of trigger points lurks there.

To find the trigger points on the inside of the thigh, have the subject lie on his or her side with the upper leg bent and out of the way. Refer now to Plate 10. Start between the two lines and work up. As you approach the three-quarter mark you will encounter a strong band of muscle in the midline. This band is made up of two muscles, the adductor magnus, spot 41, and the gracillis, spot 42. They must be elbow-pressed from either side.

While you are working in that area, check with the two marks on either side of the coccyx (tailbone). They are shown as spots 19 on Plate 5. Those two points are often responsible for spasm in the pelvis floor or levator ani, Plate 19. The levator ani is the name applied collectively to the important muscular components of the pelvis diaphragm. Spasm in the levator ani can cause frigidity, impotence, and the pain often attributed to hemorrhoids. Trigger points are put there in falls in which the subject lands either flat on the seat, as on ice, or over an obstruction, such as a curb or a board.

Press into each of those spots from the opposite side while the subject's knee is bent away from your elbow. The stretch for this area is explained on page 32.

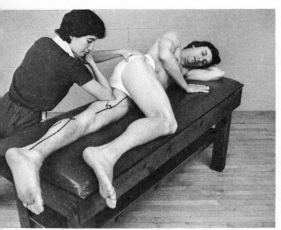

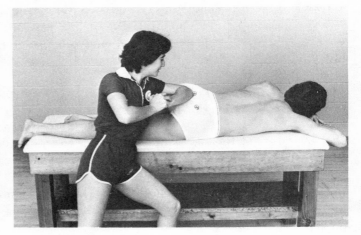

STRETCH FOR THE INSIDE OF THE UPPER LEG

When you have finished work on the inside of the upper leg, bring the subject's heel up as close to the buttocks as possible. Press the leg open and down toward the table. Stabilize the pelvis by pressing down at the same time on the near side of the pelvis. Press down and hold for three seconds. Release and repeat three more times.

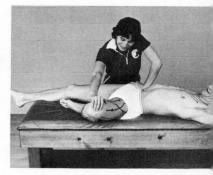

STRETCH FOR THE CENTER LINE OF THE LEG

After doing the front of the leg, have the subject move to the edge of the table and drop the leg just worked over the side. The operator pulls the foot toward the head of the table to stretch. Go gently at first, and at full stretch use the easy-bounce technique rather than static stretch. In other words do not set up opposition in the muscle, just ease it into compliance with rhythmic pulls.

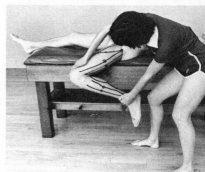

STRETCH FOR THE OUTSIDE OF THE LEG

Here, you can use the cross-leg stretch (page 33), which works for both the gluteus medius and the outer aspect of the leg.

The Lower Leg

In all probability the knee will already be much better, but there are still three sides of the lower leg to do.

Reach across the body to work on the far leg. You will be coming down the line that begins at spot 43 on the tibialis anterior (see Plate 9). This muscle contributes greatly to good balance and freedom from pain in cases of flat feet, provided it is clear of trigger points. You will be sliding between the muscle and the long shin bone, the tibia.

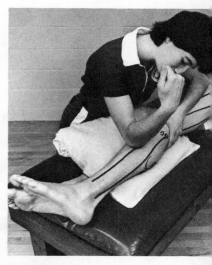

To get at the inside of the lower leg, have the subject on his or her side with the knee of the leg to be worked, bent. Starting at spot 44 (see Plate 7), run down the inside of the front on the medial side of the tibia, the long bone of the lower leg. The stretch for both sides of the leg comes from foot action.

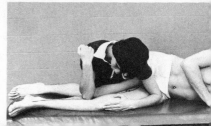

STRETCH FOR LOWER LEG PLUS STIFF AND PAINFUL ANKLES

People with stiff and painful ankles often don't even know that there is a painfree way to be. If they are young they don't know what to call this problem. If they are old they have "arthritis." Give most of it the right name, and let's get rid of it. The name: trigger points (check under The Classic Greek Foot in Chapter 6).

After your lower legs have been worked, do the following stretch exercises *often*.

1. *Pronation.* Point the toe downward as far as possible and hold for a slow count of three. Relax.
2. *Dorsiflexion.* Pull the toes upward and hold for a slow count of three.
3. *Inward rotation.* Rotate the foot inward, but don't turn the knee. Hold for three.
4. *Outward rotation.* Rotate the foot outward but don't turn the knee. Hold for three.

Those four movements make up a set. Do four sets often, and during every TV commercial.

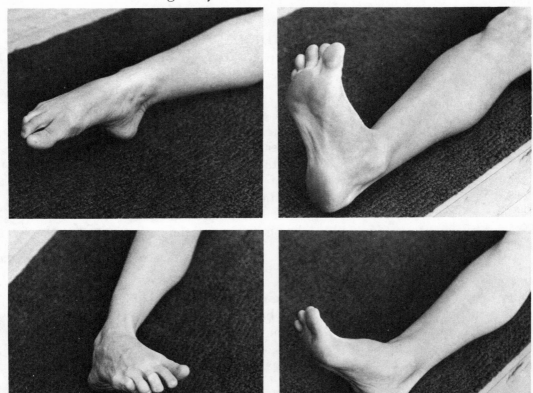

RELIEF FOR HURTING FEET

There is no age limit for hurting feet, and not much fun in life for those who have them. Check on Plate 11 and you will see a number of circles where trigger points are apt to be in feet. Use your Bodo on yourself if you work alone, but try to get a friend to help. Detrigger your feet as much as possible using the same hunting technique used around the eyes, pressing with your Bodo or finger at intervals a finger width apart. When you find a tender spot, hold for seven seconds. Try the instep first, then the outer and inner aspects of the foot, and finally the sole.

After your have detriggered your feet, do the stretches for the foot, which are the same as those for the lower leg, in the previous section.

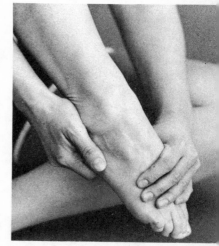

FOOT MASSAGE AND EXERCISES

Feet are often overworked, and because of confining shoes, high heels, and trigger points, they are victims of poor circulation. After detriggering your feet, you should give them both exercise and massage. To see what a difference this makes, first do only one foot and then compare it with the other.

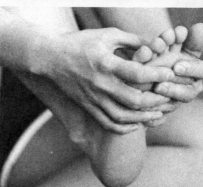

The Arch

Place the fingers of the left hand flat over the toes of the right foot with the thumb under the instep. Press the toes down to increase the arch of the foot. Alternate this exercise with the press-up.

Press-up

Place both hands under the ball of the foot and pull up as far as possible. Alternate with the arch exercise for four sets.

Twist-in

Twist the foot under as far as possible trying to point the sole toward the ceiling. This stretches the outside of both foot and ankle.

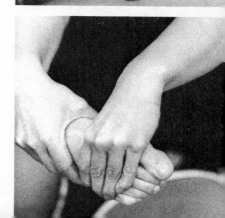

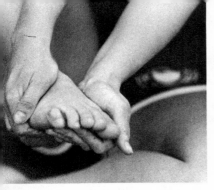

Twist-out

Grasp the foot in both hands and press down with the hand on the inside of the foot and pull up with the hand on the outside of the foot. This stretches the inner side of both foot and ankle. Alternate a twist-in with a twist-out four times.

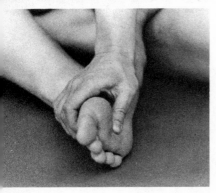

Toe Spread

Grasp the foot with both hands, placing the thumbs on top and the fingers underneath. First, spread the toes wide. Then, as though your toes were webbed, continue to separate them by pressing your thumbs against your fingers through the flesh of the toes. Spend about one minute on each foot in this manner.

Ball-Press

Place the fingers of one hand on the upper surface of the foot and the thumb on the ball. Press the thumb hard against the ball of the foot in small circles as though you were trying to loosen the bones in the foot. Spend at least one or even two minutes on each foot in this manner.

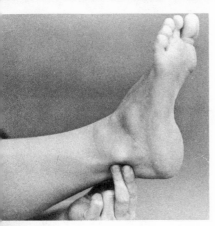

Heel-Cord Relaxer

Tight heel cords lead to fatigue, the possibility of a torn Achilles tendon, and ultimately to the old person's inflexible walk. Place the fingers on one side of the heel cord and the thumb on the other. Start at the heel and move the cord back and forth from side to side as you slowly move your hand up the leg. Repeat this action four or five times, trying to relax the foot and ankle consciously as well as manually.

By the time you have completed this foot massage, your feet will feel pleasantly warm and flexible. This is because you have worked over muscles, which improves circulation and readies your feet for the exercises to follow.

Soleus, Gastroc, and Heel-Cord Stretch

Stand with your feet parallel and heels flat on the floor. Keeping your seat tucked under, bend your knees as far as they will go while the heels are still down. At this point, bounce in short, easy bounces aiming to stretch the gastrocs, soleus, and Achilles tendon a little at a time. Bounce ten times, go on to another exercise and then later, return for another go.

Heel-Cord Stretch Continued

Stand on a book, box, or low stair with insteps and heels free in the air. Press the heels down in short bounces, ten to a set. Alternate this exercise with any other foot exercise and repeat twice more. Never waste the chance when you have to climb stairs to do a few heel-cord stretches.

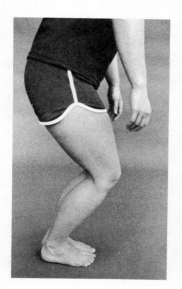 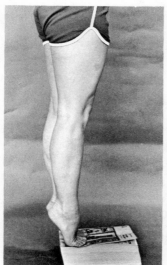 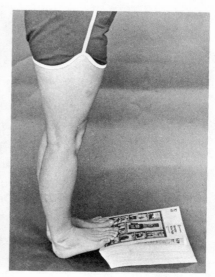

Instep Stretch

This exercise is a bit more difficult. Don't force it. Rest on hands and knees with insteps flat on the floor. Raise yourself up onto the tops of the toes increasing the arch. Drop back to the knee-rest position and repeat four or five times. After this becomes easy, bounce gently on your insteps three times before coming to rest. This exercise improves ankle flexibility, athletic performance, and even the walking and running gaits.

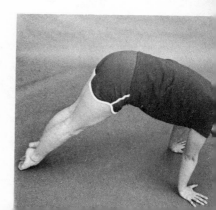

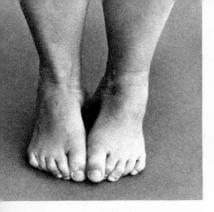

Roll-Out

Start with the feet parallel and flat on the floor. Roll onto the outer edges of the feet and curl the toes. Be sure that the toes touch in front and the heels in back. Roll back to the flat-foot position. Alternate this exercise with the toe lift.

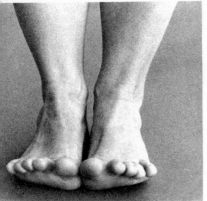

Toe Lift

From the flat-foot position raise the toes but be sure to keep the ball of the foot flat on the floor. Do six sets of toe lifts alternating with six roll-outs. These improve both the strength and flexibility of the feet and ankles.

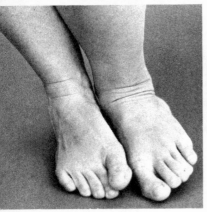

Edging

Start with feet parallel and flat on the floor. Bend both knees, keeping the pelvis tucked under. Shift both knees to the right so that the feet roll over onto their right edges. Without straightening the legs, shift the knees to the left and roll onto their left edges. Do eight shifts to a set and three sets. This is an excellent exercise for increased ankle flexibility and foot strength.

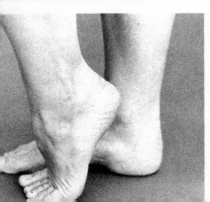

Heel Lifts

Start with the feet parallel and flat. Raise the left heel but keep the ball of the foot and the toes *flat* on the floor. The break in the foot comes just behind the toes. At first make the separate movements carefully with one foot and then the other. Later, you can pretend to march in place, alternating one foot in rhythm with the other. Start with 20 and work up to 50. Good for strength, flexibility, balance, and control.

Toe Rises

Start with the feet flat and parallel. Tighten abdominal, seat, and thigh muscles, and rise *slowly* to the toes. Lower *slowly*. Count one the first time you rise and count one for the descent. The second time take two counts to reach the peak and two to drop back to the floor. The third time take three counts and so on up to eight. Then reverse the order starting with eight and going down to one. Increases strength and balance. (If your balance wavers perhaps you have a long second toe. See under The Classic Greek Foot in Chapter 6.)

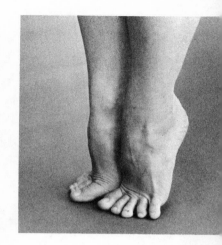

This foot section is a must for walkers, joggers, athletes, and people in occupations requiring standing. It will be helpful after a session of sport or after you have stood for a long time. If you suffer from aching feet or legs, use it daily until there is no pain.

THE CHEST MUSCLES AND PAIN

The chest muscles, the pectoralis major and minor, are a veritable hornet's nest of trigger points. If you break a rib you will put trigger points in the pectoralis. If you break your collarbone you will put trigger points in the pects. If someone punches your breastbone a good one or you bang it on the steering wheel when you can't stop in traffic, you will put trigger points in the pects. If you have menstrual cramps or a baby you can put trigger points in your pects. If you have a bad heart you will have trigger points in your pects. And for sure, if you fall forward onto your arms, or have a shoulder separation or an elbow injury, or sit over a desk you will have trigger points in the pects.

And what does that mean? It means you can have upper back pain and never know where it is coming from. It means that if you have angina it will be more painful than the next fellow's. It means that when you have menstrual cramps, medicine won't work. It means you can have a "tennis elbow" even though you don't own a racquet. It means you can have a long run of corking headaches and stiff necks, and get round-shouldered as well. One cannot ignore the pectoralis major and minor.

Asthma, emphysema, and sports are very hard on the chest muscles. Straining for breath lights up trigger points,

115

which throw muscles into spasm and make the chest less flexible. The posture assumed by the basketball player when arms are extended and shoulders rounded is not helpful. The extreme contractions demanded by the butterfly stroke in swimming, the necessity to control a horse's reins while maintaining an erect posture, the closed position of the putter, the unilateral shoulder work done in racquet sports, the closed shoulders of the oarsman, and the torque required of the batter—all put trigger points into the pects.

Football does a good share of its damage before the game, while the boys are building tight, bulky muscles with never a thought to flexibility. Then during the mayhem that is called a game the inflexible chest muscles result in torn shoulder muscles because they are incapable of normal stretch. Jogging tenses both chest and shoulders often via tense hands and arms.

Occupations contribute to chest-muscle problems and add the problem of insufficient oxygen intake as straps of shortened muscle fiber lash the chest tight in an ungiving embrace. The roundbacked and often fibrositic typist, dentist, surgeon, architect, jeweler, seamstress, and press operator all shorten the fibers in chest muscles even as they overstretch the weakened upper back muscles.

Emotions play havoc with chest muscles. The desire to be someplace else, which can begin when early childhood is less than lovely, pulls the shoulders protectively forward and up while the head sinks down into the collar. Every muscle involved becomes tight and inflexible. If this is maintained long enough we soon see what we call "the forward head." Since the spine is constantly rounded and since the head, which is attached to the spine, holds the neck in a curve and forces the face and eyes into the same rounding curve, the sufferer has trouble seeing what's ahead. To rectify matters the face is then lifted, which further strains neck, back, shoulders, and chest. Aside from being a poor substitute for a direct gaze, this strain will ultimately cause pain and can lead to other (often unexplained) troubles such as jaw pain, stiff necks, the stiff and painful shoulder syndrome, earache, and even, because the conduit called the neck is so much affected, poor circulation to the head.

Disease affects the chest muscles. A good example is the person who has angina pectoris, a heart condition that comes under the heading of disease. *Angina* means "a spasmodic chok-

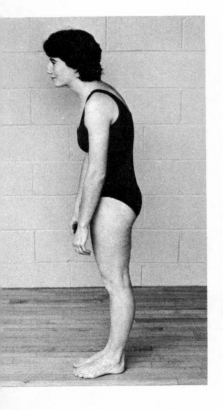

116

ing, or suffocative, pain." *Pectoris* refers to the breast or chest. The disease lays down trigger points in the chest, and when it attacks it not only contributes its own pain but signals the trigger points to fire, which throws the muscles into spasm and causes even more pain. If you have an angina sufferer in the family, ask your doctor if you may erase the trigger points when all is well. You would be able to make the agony less when it is not.

CLEARING TRIGGER POINTS FROM THE CHEST MUSCLES

To take trigger points out of the pectoralis major is easy. Start with the subject lying supine and begin at spot 22, shown on Plate 6 in Appendix 1. Move at one-inch intervals across the chest toward the sternum. The sternum is the breastbone, found in the front of the chest and to which the first through the seventh ribs are attached. When there are trigger points found almost anywhere in the pectoralis major, there will be some on both sides of the sternum. If you find them on one side of the chest you will find them on the other side as well.

After crossing the chest on the spot 22 line, go down to spot 21 and work across. On males there is no interference from the breast, so you can move right across doing the line across the chest from spot 20. On females you do have interference, and you may also have to contend with the fear of bruising. Explain that (1) you won't bruise, and (2) that the breast gland is moveable. Then move it out of your way.

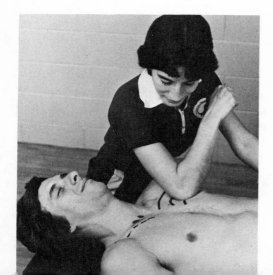

117

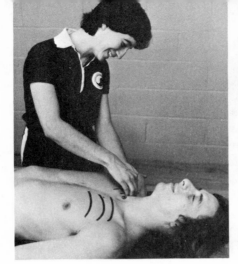

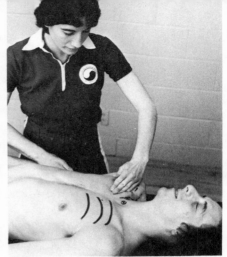

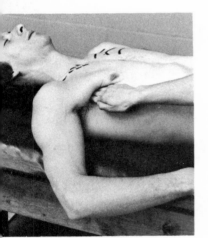

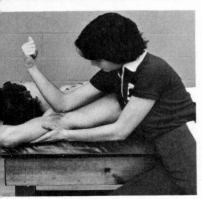

Spots 24 and 25 represent the beginning of two lines, one above and one below the clavicle, or collarbone. To clear the top of the collarbone, reach into the hollow between the bone and the neck with curved fingers and pull down against the bone. Begin at the sternum and work out to the shoulder. Do both sides.

For the underside of the collarbone, press up into the bone and work again out to the shoulder in each direction.

Then using the wraparound technique (page 52) place your fingers under the bone and wrap around over the bone.

Next you will need to clear the pectoralis minor, at spot 23. This muscle attaches to the third, fourth, and fifth ribs in front and to the scapula in back. See again how connected the back is to the front and vice versa? Slide under the pectoralis muscle as deep as possible and press against the ribs. Also make sure you have cleared the scapula by doing grid D on Plate 5. Any damage to the shoulder at any time may well affect the pectoralis minor and translate to chest pain. Now who would connect an old football injury to the shoulder, or a clowning bang on the upper back at one's fifteenth reunion, with what feels like angina?

We are not quite through with the front of the chest until we have looked at the axilla, shown on Plate 18. This small pyramidal area between the upper lateral part of the chest and the medial side of the arm includes, in addition to the armpit, many nerves, a large number of lymph nodes, fat and areolar tissue—and some of the most painful trigger points extant. Plant your elbow almost anywhere in that area and the subject will tell you they are there, loudly and emphatically. There is no particular spot or line to work on in the axilla. Trigger points can be anywhere. Just be sure to cover the field. Pain causes sweating, and sweating areas are slippery. Cover the axilla with a washcloth soaked with cool water and wrung out, or one with a bit of alcohol poured into it. It prevents slipping as well as embarrassment to the subject. It also feels better to the questing elbow!

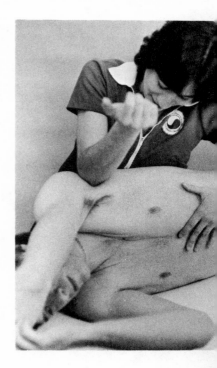

The latissimus dorsi must also be investigated as a part of clearing the chest. Refer here to grid E shown on Plate 5. The subject lies on his or her side with arms raised and extended. Begin at the top near the armpit and work down the muscle at the usual one-inch intervals. Include the entire grid in your search.

This muscle, like the sternocleidomastoid, has many jobs and is therefore at multiple risk. Its job is to extend, adduct, and rotate the arm. Any damage to the spine, the ilium, the ribs, or the scapula can mean referred pain to the arm. Put the other way, any damage to the arm could refer pain to the back, both upper and lower. Do the following exercises after detriggering the chest.

SNAP AND STRETCH EXERCISE FOR THE LATISSIMUS DORSI

Stand with feet apart and arms bent at shoulder level. Without lowering the level of the arms, snap the elbows back to stretch the chest muscles on the count of one. Return hands to starting position in front of the chest on the count of two. On three, fling arms wide *at shoulder level*. On four return to the starting position.

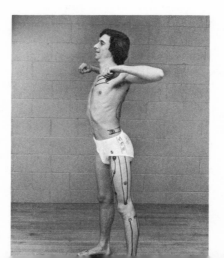

119

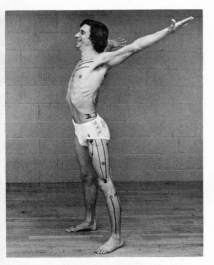

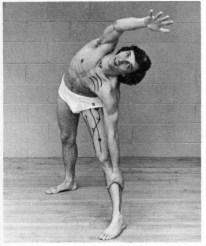

To make this exercise pay off for the axilla as well as the latissimus dorsi, make two slight changes. Snap the elbows back as before, but on the fling, raise the arms up one foot as in the illustration and face the palms forward (not illustrated). Return to start. Do eight of each kind, level and with arms raised one foot.

LATERAL OVERHEAD REACH

This exercise is specifically a stretch for axilla and latissimus dorsi—and a must for people who work with arms tight to their sides, lift weights, drive cars, buses, trucks or heavy equipment, and for dentists and surgeons.

Stand with feet apart and place the left hand on the lower leg just below the knee. Stretch the right arm to the left side over the head. Bring the hand in to cover the ear. Reach the arm out again as far as possible. Four to a side is a set. Do four sets.

PAIN IN THE ARMS AND HANDS

I woke one morning with my shoulder and elbow aching and my fingers in a state we call "numbling," which means they are halfway between numb and tingling. Probably I had slept on it most of the night. From the feel of things I was suffering all the symptoms of "bursitis" and "tennis elbow" with a little "arthritis" thrown in. What to do? I had to be in Chicago that evening. By noon I was still numbling so I called in the troops. I was like the shoemaker's child, the last one to seek myotherapy.

Look at Plates 16 and 17 in Appendix 1 as you read what follows. You will then understand why you should not look for the cause of hand pain in your hand or wrist pain in your wrist (unless, of course, either has just been gashed, smashed, or otherwise acutely "insulted").

Arms and hands bring many trigger points home to roost, not only in themselves but in the surrounding areas—chest, upper back, neck, jaw, face, and head. Weight lifters, boxers, wrestlers, football players—and piano players—hurt their arms. Dentists and dental hygienists and violinists hurt their arms. Weavers, knitters, and crocheters and those who drive cars,

120

trucks, and tractors hurt their hands, and arms. Arms can be strained with heavy work or during repetitive work.

I used to practice on a violin (I didn't say play one). After about two hours I'd get a sliver of pain starting about four inches down the back of my left shoulder. Later when I practiced the piano, same thing. When I began writing, same thing. Then we discovered myotherapy. The spot causing the trouble was found as expected at the point of the pain (the trapezius), but its fellow conspirator, the one setting off the spasm, was at the spot numbered 76 on Plate 17. That muscle, the extensor carpi radialis longus, extends and raises the wrist joint. All violinists and dentists have trigger points in that muscle. And those have a couple of close friends at spots 75, 77, and 79.

If you look closely at Plate 17, the arm, you will see immediately how trigger points in the chest and shoulder, the armpit area, or the upper and lower arm could affect your hands, and vice versa. And your hands can also affect your neck, jaw, face, and head.

With that in mind, give heed to what you do with your hands. Do you clench your fists? Do you bang on can openers to force them through the tops of cans? Do you do endless small hand work? Do you fidget? Do you twist off jar tops that require great strength? Do you ride horses, which requires strength in hands, arms, and upper back? Do you use a single lever to operate heavy equipment? Do you play a lot of handball? Do you squeeze the handle of your racquet? Do you practice long hours at an instrument? drive long hours in a car? I'm not suggesting that you give up anything (except banging on can openers). I do suggest that you have someone clear your arms, hands, upper back, and chest of trigger points (in that order) on a regular basis to prevent pain and trouble now or later.

THE ARM

Elbow Below the Joint

Have the subject lie supine with arm flat on the table palm down. Start at spot 75 (see Plate 17) on the brachioradialis. Note that the muscle appears fairly narrow. Go down its inner edge at one-inch intervals into the wrist, pressing toward the median line of the arm. Next, start at spot 76, the extensor carpi

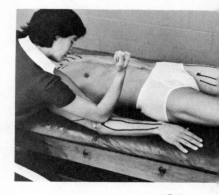

radialis longus. You will catch the other edge of the brachioradialis as you go down that line into the wrist. *Attention those who are said to have carpal tunnel syndrome!* We have found very often this is the muscle causing the pain. Note also where its lower attachment is, spot 78. Be very sure to de-fuse that one. Use the knuckle or a Bodo.

SHOULDER ROTATIONS

To stretch the arm after detriggering, stand, resting most of your weight on the right foot. Rotate the right arm in a counter-clockwise direction as far as you can and watch your thumb come around as you exhale fully. Then turn your arm in the opposite direction as far as you can, breathing in. Start with four to each side and then do eight together. Do three sets. This exercise improves the shoulder range and stretches and strengthens the arms and upper back and chest muscles.

Try to include this exercise as part of your daily routine—when leaving the office, while doing chores in the house, or after going to the bathroom. Anything will do so long as it reminds you to loosen your shoulders and arms.

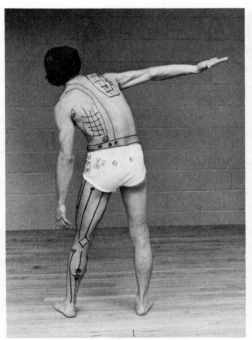 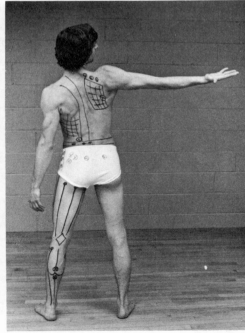

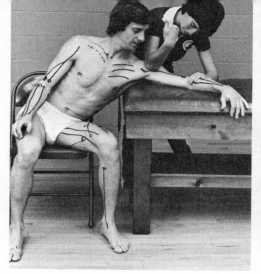
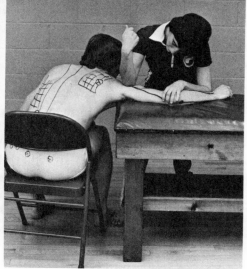

Elbow Above the Joint

Have the subject sit on a chair with the arm stretched out on the table with palm down. Start at spot 79 (see Plate 17), which denotes the brachialis line. Work at half-inch intervals to a point midway between elbow and shoulder. Stop at spot 80, the lower edge of the deltoid muscle.

The deltoid resembles a small cape covering the top of the arm. You want to work up first one side of the muscle to the shoulder and then up the other side. When that is completed return to spot 79 for a second sortie up the brachialis line to spot 80. This time, however, your concern is with the biceps in the front of the arm and the triceps at the back. To trap trigger points in the biceps press toward the front of the arm. To reach those in the triceps press toward the back.

Arm Palm Up

Have the subject lie prone with the back of the arm on the table and palm up. Start near the elbow at spot 81 on the pronator teres, shown on Plate 16. This is a "starter" muscle. That means it is a small muscle that is responsible for starting action that will be taken over by larger, stronger muscles. A trigger point in this muscle means a poor start, a late start, or maybe no start. The pronator teres should always be considered at risk when the sport, occupation, or habit calls for a great many starts, say a dental hygienist cleaning teeth all day every day. Go down the line started at the pronator teres into the wrist.

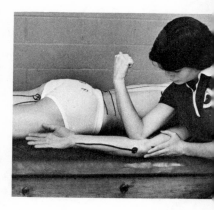

Spot 82, on the flexor carpi ulnaris, begins the outer line. As you work next to the belly of the muscle, press both inward and outward as well as straight down toward the table.

123

Above the Joint
Start again at the pronator teres (see Plate 16), this time working upward. The inside line will press into the biceps. The outside line will press into the triceps. The middle line will allow you to press straight down into the triceps. Work along the outer edge of the arm, up into the deltoid, and on the inside edge into the teres major in the upper back, to spot 12.

THE HAND

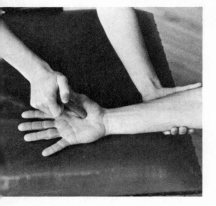

Like the foot, the hand can house trigger points almost any-where. The three most likely to be present are shown at spots 83, 84, and 85 on Plates 16 and 17. The one most likely to give trouble is number 83. Use your knuckle or a Bodo to locate them. The technique for clearing the fingers after you have done the arms and hands is called a four-way squeeze.

Four-Way Squeeze
There are 14 phalanges (finger bones), and each one has the potential to give you a headache, swollen fingers and knuckles, or a painful hand, wrist, or even arm.

Hold the subject's hand, palm down against your palm, and squeeze the two sides of the first phalange of the first finger very gently at first, between your thumb and finger. Then re-volve your thumb and finger to squeeze the front and back. Move down to the second and then the third phalange. Rarely is there trouble in the third phalange; you will find it often in the second and first. The hands of arthritics offer the greatest challenge and reward, but imagine the thrill of returning a functioning finger to a concert musician! Remember, when working with hands the fingers come last. The shoulders and everything in between come first.

EXERCISES FOR THE HAND
One would think hands get exercise enough, but they don't; they get work and often overwork. After detriggering your hands and arms, do exercises to strengthen and stretch hands and fingers. Be sure to stretch them after any work.

Here are some simple exercises:

squeezing a rubber ball
stretching a rubber band
wringing a washcloth

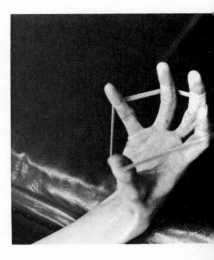

Stretch Exercises for Hands

Hold the palm of the left hand up and then cover the fingers of the left hand with those of the right. Extend the left arm straight forward as the right hand stretches the fingers down and back. Return to start and do four. Repeat with other hand.

Repeat the same exercise stretching each individual finger. Do the stretch after the other exercises for hands and arms and always after a warm bath—even after hand washing.

Ignore no pain connected with your hands. The cause doesn't just fade away but lies in wait for years. Look at the hands of old people and see what the accumulation of years and trigger points can do. You need good hands. Take care of yours.

ATHLETES, WEEKEND SPORTSMEN, AND THEIR PAINS

Most sports injuries are sustained by comparatively young people who are comparatively healthy. To us at this institute this means that the muscles are in comparatively good condition and for the most part free of spasm. A climate of tension, however, can be found wherever there is competition, and that means from the most active sport to the least active. The young executive trying to beat out his competition on the links with the boss watching is in equal danger (as far as climate is concerned) with the football player trying for a reputation on Saturday's gridiron.

The more strenuous the sport, however (the climate being equal), the greater the chance for injury. Sports injuries go by many names, meaning many different conditions: meniscus, spurs, chondromalacia, carpal tunnel syndrome, bursitis, myositis, tendinitis, and many others. We feel, however (and our experience in the treatment room has shown), that most of this is really muscle spasm caused by trigger points laid down

125

when the muscles were "insulted." And with athletes, there's plenty of opportunity for that to happen.

Darlene Jones, a trainer who has studied with us, has been getting 97 percent success in as few as one or two sessions in the training room at Lehigh University. Other trainers are turning in similar scores. We feel that this may have a bearing on the future care of athletes, even in the prevention of injury.

A poll was taken of 1,000 serious runners. Those are the ones who actually run, not talk about it. An astonishing two thirds of them had suffered injuries serious enough to lay them up for two weeks. Now how could such a gentle sport as jogging lay anyone up for *any* time unless there is more to the story than meets the macadam. Of course there is. Why the accident happens is usually simple—trigger points. The trigger points may have been there since hopscotch, Little League, and jump-rope days, but it takes the constant pounding on a hard surface to activate them. No self-respecting horse person would trot a horse on the road. Bad for their valuable legs.

While the seasoned athlete as well as the would-be athlete can damage almost any part of the body in the heat of competition, one joint seems to be at particular risk, the knee. It is a complex, rather poorly constructed joint which can cope with the stresses put upon it only if the muscles protecting it as well as activating it are strong. Keep in mind that a muscle harboring a trigger point causing spasm is not as strong as it should be or seems to be.

One could blame the tremendous number of knee injuries on the fact that we are a nation that takes its first step, after crawling, onto wheels. It's understandable that weekend athletes would have knee problems, but look at some other people who have injured knees—people with some of the best knees in the country: O. J. Simpson, Phil Esposito, Julius Erving, Billy Cunningham, Wilt Chamberlain, Larry Csonka, and Joe Namath. Those men were all prepared for their sport. They had the best trainers and the best coaches. It's a pretty safe bet, however, that neither they nor those in charge of their health and safety knew much about what trigger points can do, how to find them, or how to extinguish them.

With the best athletes in the country in so much danger of injury it is little wonder that the average jogger, Saturday morning touch football addict, weekend skier, and players of softball, basketball, and volleyball complains of "trick knees," "shinsplints," "bursitis," "tennis elbow," "tendinitis," "spurs," and an aching back.

Any damage to a leg, at any time, and from any form of punishment—a torn muscle, muscle fatigue, a hairline fracture, or even such a simple anomaly as the long second toe—can lay down trigger points that will come back to strike one day.

Probably the most talked-about injury today is tennis elbow. It is said to be an inflammation of the tendon that joins the muscle of the forearm to the outside of the elbow. In our work we find that the word *inflammation* is applied all too often, and that most of the time the term *trigger points* would be more apt.

Elbows, like knees, are often put under severe strain in sports. "Little League elbow" applies to the pain suffered by children playing a lot of baseball and not much else. Later when those children grow up and switch to tennis, "tennis elbow" will be the name given the same condition.

Since I have been an athlete all my life I realize nobody is going to keep an athlete from playing his or her game. And nobody can stop the athlete from picking up trigger points. But you can take charge of your own training. And you can find your own trigger points and erase them—*before* they ruin either your muscles or your score.

Jenny Fisher, who is 16, says, "I won my first 'A' NELTA [New England Lawn Tennis Association] sanctioned tournament and I owe it to myotherapy (and my mother of course).

"First of all, because of rain, the first two matches were moved indoors on hard courts, which really tightened up my legs. My mother did the trigger point work on my leg muscles after each of these matches. That kept them from cramping.

"The last two days of the tournament I had to play two matches, the semifinals and the finals. I was really nervous and tight before the semifinals, because I was playing the number two seed, so my mom did my arms and shoulders which relaxed me. I asked her to do my shoulders and arms again just before the finals because it kept them very flexible, which I needed for serving. I didn't double fault once in the finals.

"The myotherapy helped relieve both the physical and mental tension for me."

Athletes, like almost everybody else, are confused about the causes of their injuries, aches, and pains. They think the

127

triggering mechanism—the fast ball, the top spin, or the golfer's slice—actually caused the sudden agonizing pain. Too often, like Randy Gardner in the 1980 Winter Olympics, they pull up lame at the critical moment—never realizing that the condition had been in the muscles for months, possibly years. Check with the sports chart in Appendix 4 of this book, and find out which muscles are most at risk in which sport. See to it that those muscles are clear of trigger points *before* you compete. (A Sunday golf tournament, tennis match, marathon, water meet—all are competition just as much as the Saturday pro game.) Then follow up *after* the game with seeking massage (see under Seeking Massage later in this chapter) to find out what kind of damage that game did—and erase it.

IMMEDIATE MOBILIZATION

Immediate mobilization doesn't count for much unless you are a wilderness backpacker, a cross country skier, a professional dancer, a professional actor, a professional musician, a professional lecturer, a professional TV performer—in other words, a professional anybody who has to be in there today at ten, two, or eight. Or a person who leaves civilization for greener, icier, snowier, colder, hotter, or wilder climates. Then you need to know.

In the case of the professional injured just down the street, the X-ray will probably be negative. He can't walk, but he may have to.

In the case of the person hurt in the wilderness, he has to get back to civilization either under his own steam or on someone else's back. And the former is much to be preferred. It would, in either instance, gimping professional or limping backpacker, be helpful to be able to do what has to be done, given that you don't have a choice.

Fluori-Methane, the coolant spray, is one answer. If a bone is broken, the spray won't help. You will hurt as much after using it as before, or worse. Figure you are busted and act accordingly. If the spray does help, you are most probably sprained.

A sprain is defined as a temporary dislocation in which some of the fibers of a supporting ligament are torn, but the continuity of the ligament remains intact. In other words, there are minute tears with an accompanying leakage of blood into the tissue surrounding the joint, but function is not disrupted. In still other words, the joint could work if it didn't hurt.

Anyone who has ever sprained an ankle knows that after the initial wrenching pain it is quite possible to walk back to camp or the showers, or to return up the cellar stairs. It's after you *stop* walking that the real pain sets in. Why? The answer starts with the "insulted" muscle which now (and quite possibly before the accident) has trigger points in residence. The trigger points cause the muscles around the joint to go into spasm, which adds even more pain to the injured ankle. Within minutes of the accident there will be spasm as high up the leg as the knee, and this produces another complication. Muscles in acute spasm act like clamps on vessels. The blood and fluid leaking into the tissue cannot be transported away from the area, and swelling begins. Swelling causes pressure and more pain. Moving the joint becomes impossible. In addition, circulation *to* the injured area is now impaired, which retards healing. This whole unhealthy situation can be altered in a matter of minutes—the sooner the better.

First, locate and extinguish the trigger points starting in the hip and groin. Many trigger points in adjacent areas are alerted by injury and called to participate in producing spasm. Work down the leg to the ankle, but not into it. Skip to the foot and find all you can. By the time you are ready for the ankle, the swelling should be somewhat reduced. Hunt gently around the ankle and erase any trigger points you find.

The next step is the stretching. Use the ankle stretches in the section Stretch for Lower Legs Plus Stiff and Painful Ankles earlier in the chapter. Have your subject go through the series of four exercises three or four times. As he moves tentatively there will be some discomfort in the foot, ankle, or leg, depending on the injury. Spray the coolant spray along the muscle housing pain in lines about one half inch apart, always in the same direction. In the illustration, a marker has been used to show you how to spray. If the spray is not available use the *corner* of an ice cube.

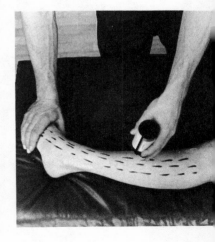

It is also necessary to squeeze the still accumulating blood and fluid out of the injured area, thus preventing swelling, pressure, pain, and impaired circulation. This is accomplished with

129

resistance exercise. In resistance exercise, as is so often the case of myotherapy, there is a partnership between subject and therapist. The subject now provides the will and the power to put the joint through a full range of motion. The myotherapist provides the resistance that will force the muscles to work harder and thus squeeze more efficiently. The subject accepts only as much pain as is tolerable, and both people will discover that while the first round of exercises may be undertaken tentatively, strength and range will return quickly. The coolant spray or ice cube should be used liberally whenever there is pain.

Do four or five repetitions of the following resistance exercises for the ankle.

The Ankle

Pronation

Press down against a fist placed under the ball of the foot.

Dorsiflexion

Pull up against fingers placed over the instep.

Inward Rotation

Turn the foot inward against the resistance of a hand held on the inside of the foot.

Outward Rotation

Turn the foot outward against the resistance of a hand held on the outside of the foot.

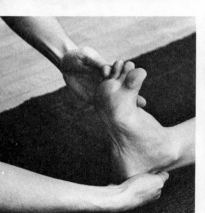

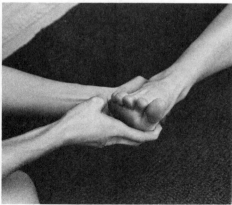

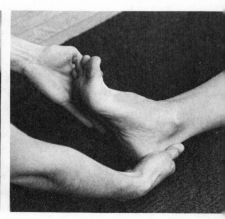

Repeat the resistance exercises for the ankle every hour the first day and every two hours the second, even if you find you can walk comparatively painlessly. If you are in the wilderness, this means every hour during the day and every two during the night. If you are in New York or Topeka and the doctor has said, "Nothing but a sprain," you can interrupt your work for a night's sleep. If your act comes on at three the next day, though, you'd better give up that night's sleep.

The Wrist

The wrist is usually not as critical in the wilderness since you don't have to walk back on it. But suppose you were a canoeist, or a cross country skier. Wrists aren't usually critical for lecturers, but supposing you are the first violinist in the Boston Symphony, or the conductor. Suppose, for example, you are Sir Laurence Olivier—or Bonnie Prudden—and the show must go on.

Go through a trigger point search starting in the armpit. Work your way down the entire arm to just above the wrist. Then tackle the hand. The wrist is last, and the swelling will be down when you reach it. The same resistance exercises are used in order to obtain full range of motion and to keep the swelling down.

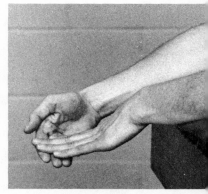

Pronation

Press downward against the resistance of your other hand pressing up.

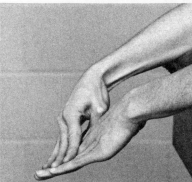

Dorsiflexion

Press upward against the resistance of your other hand pressing down.

Inward Rotation

Turn your arm on its side and press up against the resistance of your own hand pressing down.

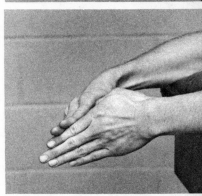

Outward Rotation

Press down against the upward pressure of your other hand.

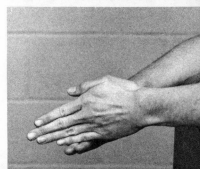

And the same goes for wrists as for ankles—*every hour.*

SEEKING MASSAGE

Seeking massage is an essential part of myotherapy. It can be used either before or after trigger point work to seek out sensitive spots still in the muscles. This can be helpful too when there isn't time to check out every muscle inch by inch. Seeking massage could be used to advantage just before the game, the night before the race, the evening after a long and tiring trip, and on a regular basis for people whose occupations strain or damage muscles constantly. It acts to reinforce myotherapy, helping muscles that have been freed of spasm to stay free. The first stage, double or loosening massage, should follow any extensive search for trigger points.

Double Massage (Loosening)

This is a kind of seeking massage but is performed by two people and is done to music. This more than quadruples the effectiveness of the work because it confuses the expectations, and even the experience of the subject counts for little. It is easy to figure out what one person is doing with two hands. It is impossible to figure out what two are doing with four, which feel like eight. Resistance is brought to an all-time low. In addition, muscles "listen" to music.

Use oil that pleases, not hand cream.

Circles

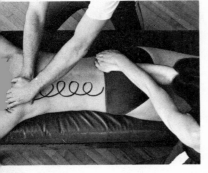

Select for your music something slightly hypnotic, something that goes on and on for the 15 minutes you will be working.

The first operator makes circular motions with both hands moving together from the waist to a point over the shoulder. The second operator, preparing to do the same thing, makes ready at the waist on the other side. Then as one leaves off the other begins. At no time are both operators' hands free of the body; one or the other is in contact at all times. Repeat according to the phrases in the music; when it says move on to another type of massage, move on.

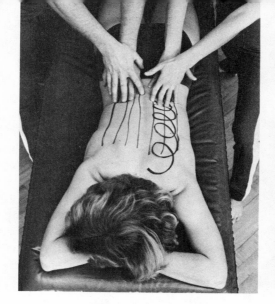
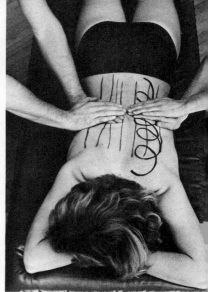

The Rake

The fingers, all sixteen of them, start at the waist and slide like a rake up the back to the shoulders. The hands then move outward and slide back down the sides to the flanks. *Keep contact.* Do four rakes.

The Smoother

Slide all four hands up both sides of the back and back down the sides. Four times or according to the music.

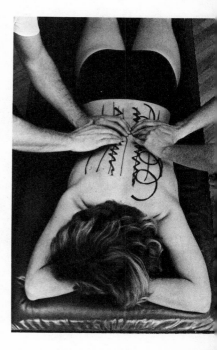

The Jiggle

The fingers of the lead hand of each operator (the one closer to the subject's shoulders) vibrate up the muscles on either side of the spine, and the second hand follows with some pressure. Slide the hands back down the sides. Do four, or as many as the music requires.

After three sets, each of which is comprised of circles, rakes, smoothers, and jiggles, move down to the legs.

The Wringer (Lower Legs)

Start the legs massage by reaching down with one hand to grasp each ankle while the other hand remains on the back. Use a wringing motion from ankle to knee, both operators doing identical motions, each to a leg. Slide the hands back down over the leg and do four times.

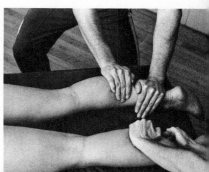

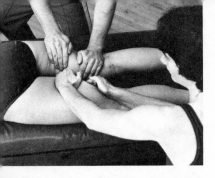

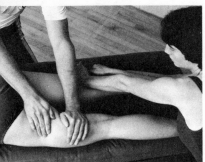

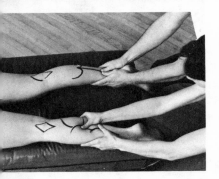

Kneading

Move on up to the thigh and knead the inner sides of the thigh. Slide the hands back down the backs of the legs to the knee. Do four times. Reach over to the outside and repeat.

Weaving

Using the thumbs as on the left leg in the illustration, smooth across the back of the lower leg from ankle to knee. Alternate thumbs. Do four times, each time sliding back down the leg along its sides.

Splitting the Gastrocs

Place both thumbs in the middle of the Achilles tendon in the back of the lower leg (see the right leg of the illustration for weaving, and press into the muscle up into the back of the knee. Do four, alternating with weaving.

Splitting the Thigh Lines

Refer here to Plate 8 in Appendix 1. Make a fist and press hard into each of the trigger point guidelines shown in the thigh. Move the fist from the knee right up to the buttocks *once* in each line. The same work can be done on the fronts and sides of the legs, and even on the arms.

Seeking

Once the massage is completed use the same technique you employed for spliting the gastrocs on the arms and all around the lower legs. If your knuckles work better for you, use them. Seeking massage is performed by one person, since you are looking for trouble spots and want the subject to concentrate on what hurts and what doesn't. Move slowly along the limb maintaining a deep and steady pressure. The subject closes his eyes and concentrates fully on the pressure. If at any time the fingers or knuckles pass over a tender spot, the subject says, "Hold it." There will be a trigger point at that spot. Stop and erase it immediately. Use knuckles on the upper legs and back, but fingers for chest and neck.

FIBROSITIS MASSAGE

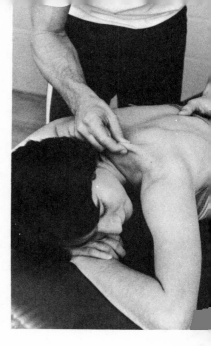

This is quite different from seeking massage, since you can see all too well the thickened areas of tissue that you are trying to eliminate. Muscles, when they are not working, are not supposed to be thick and hard. They should be soft and relaxed. Skin is not supposed to be stuck tight to the underlying tissues of the shoulders, but should be easily pulled away, like the skin on a kitten. Lori has none of the thickened tissue called "fibrositis" in her shoulders. If she did it would require the same kneading that you did on the thighs in seeking massage.

Fibrositis Arms

This is best done on yourself. Start at the elbow and knead the flesh upward with a twisting motion. When you have spent about 30 seconds on each arm do the shoulder rotations, page 122.

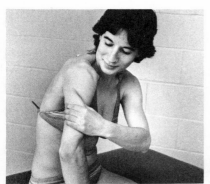 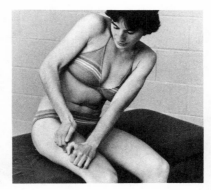

Fibrositis Thighs, Front

Do the same kneading to the front of the thighs, always working up from knee to groin. Spend a minute on each thigh.

Fibrositis "Saddle Bags"

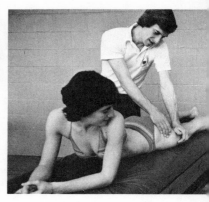

You will need help for this one and the next, the hips. Knead up the outside of the leg from the knee right up to the hip line. Two trips up the leg at one time are enough.

Fibrositis Hips

Stay inside a five-inch radius and spend roughly 15 seconds on a side.

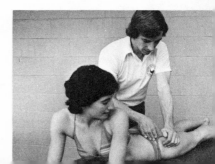

A word about fibrositis.

Fibrositis was first known by that name. It is better known to Americans by its more exotic name "cellulite." By whichever name, it is lumpy and unsightly. We believe it is caused by constant tightening when stress is present. It is found mostly on women. It contributes to shoulder and back pain and should be massaged away. Fibrositis massage hurts a lot. Start gently. Within weeks you will be able to treat it much more harshly as it gradually softens and disappears.

After fibrositis massage, do the hip and leg exercises in the exercise section of this book, Chapter 10.

Pain Related to Pregnancy And Birth—Help for Mother and Child

8

My mother's mother gave birth to six children, all of them in her own bed, leaning against a bolster with her knees bent and her feet flat on the mattress. It is said she held on to her sister's hands a lot of the time, but made no sound. It would not have been seemly. The family doctor made it for the first three babies, a midwife attended the next two, but my Aunt Marguerite, who was compulsively punctual all her life, was early for her birthday. The cook delivered her. All the babies were healthy, red, and squalling. My grandmother managed them all. And she never had a backache.

WHAT'S SO DIFFERENT TODAY?

What does all this mean? Simply that times were different then. Women were different. Life was different; and I'm not quarreling with antibiotics or improved prenatal care. Birth was normal probably because bodies were normal. Today birth is no longer normal because bodies are no longer normal. What's so different today? A lot.

First, American girls, sedentary from birth, have become weak, tense, and inflexible.

Then, too, many of them have been exposed to all forms of drugs since babyhood. I have seen first-graders come up to the teacher and say, "I'm feeling funny, can I have my Ritalin now?"

137

Ours is a drug-oriented culture. And this unfortunate state has much bearing on what is happening to children today.

Also, when we moved out of the bedroom and into the hospital, we did kind and good things to those specialists who replaced the family doctors. By lifting mothers up a foot or two we helped the OB-GYN doctors, but they let their two specialties get mixed up. Gynecology treats the diseases of the genital tract in women. The practice of that specialty requires a table, hard and narrow, at the lower end sprouting two metal stirrups for supporting the legs of the woman being examined in a spread position. If the woman has trigger points in her groin, legs, or back, she may well get a backache and leg cramps.

Now what probably happened was that for delivery purposes the doctors liked their higher table better than the back-breaking (for them) bed, so they simply had the last stages of labor transferred from beds to tables.

The trouble was and continues to be that this is the wrong position for delivery. No primitive mother could deliver herself of a baby lying flat on her back with her legs in the air. She has to be curled in a half sitting position, or squatting. That way the bady can slide down and out with nobody the worse for it.

With the accepted position today the baby has to climb over the taut perineum, and since all too often it is being assisted by forceps or speed-up drugs, the perineum tears. That's messy, of course, and somewhere along the line someone decided that making a nice clean incision (whether it's needed or not) before the baby came would be neater. The potential for laying down trigger points in all this seems endless.

Of course, there are two sides to every coin. OB-GYN doctors may have been responsible for that damn table on which women lie with legs and arms strapped as for an execution, but the American woman is responsible for the fact that she is not fit physically to birth a baby.

Let's start with drugs, because in the vernacular, that's where it's at today.

It was once thought that the placenta acted as a screening device and could protect babies from anything ingested by the mother that might be harmful. It's just not so, and our best and most well-known doctors have been shouting it from the hospital tops. If a drug is administered in sufficient quantity to either relieve pain or induce labor, it will be found in significant amounts in the fetus. What's a significant amount? The mother, who probably weighs in at 150, is getting the dose, the baby at 6½ pounds wringing wet is right there, too. Think about it!

All the following substances cross the placenta and affect the baby.

Antithyroid medications cross and affect the fetal thyroid-pituitary axis.

Barbiturates cross at all stages of gestation. Want a zonked baby?

All narcotics used in labor cross and may produce depression in newborns.

All inhalation narcotics cross and depress newborns.

Regional anesthetics readily cross.

Thiazide diuretics cross. Who-sis isn't even here yet and we are meddling with its plumbing.

Coumadin and other anticoagulants cross, and what happens when a tiny person's blood can't coagulate?

When drugs cross the placenta, or when they lower the mother's blood-gas exchange to the fetus, guess who suffers—Little Who-sis.

The morning I was slated for a cesarean because of my ski accident, a nurse came into the room. I was hyper with hidden terror. I was given a shot, two shots, three shots. No one told me what was in any of them. If you ever let anyone do that to you now, you will deserve what happens. I still didn't calm down. You know the type, merrily talking. I got another shot. I was wheeled to the operating room and anesthetized before "prepping" (they learned that technique from the Spanish Inquisition). Sometime later I learned that my first child had been born blue and not breathing. Why? Anesthetics for a 150-pound woman hit five pounds, three ounces, of new humanity.

Why is this happening? Strong, well set up, healthy women are a rarity in America today. Most who come in for delivery are weak, lacking in muscle tone and endurance, and many are accustomed to drugs. So are the doctors.

There is also "convenience." Convenience foods, convenience apartments, convenience of the customers, and convenience of the hospital. If Little Who-sis still feels he has some

139

finishing touches to wind up, too bad. All the signs say he can make it in this none-too-perfect world, and somebody has vacation plans, wants a baby born on her own birthday or Mama's, wants to leave Monday on a business trip, has a full schedule next week. So get set, Who-sis, here it comes—the hurry-up medicine. And here, too, comes the opportunity for lots of trigger points to settle in mother and baby.

There is another way to hustle the laggard, and that's by breaking the "bag of waters," that is, rupturing the embryonic membrane with a blunt instrument. Now Who-sis has no cushion for its little head which is being used as a battering ram. If we combine deflation of head cushion with hurry-up potions there can be very real trouble, including disalignment of the parietal bones of the baby's skull. This can happen in a normal birth, but it happens twice as often in induced labor.

Having had two cesarean sections because of that ski accident, I have a lot to say against them unless absolutely necessary. First, it takes a lot more out of you than just a baby. Second, the scar is not only unsightly, it can harbor trigger points. Third, the mother is in no shape to accept the baby when she is needed, which is immediately after birth. The first 24 hours are crucial. Fourth, read *Touching* by Ashley Montagu and you will discover that the gentle and not so gentle massage provided by the normal birthing process is designed to get the baby's systems into GO. Cesarean babies have all sorts of problems with their systems, from breathing to digestion. Cesarean babies don't look like they have just gone five rounds with Smokey Bear, but they can yell for months with colic. So why am I telling you this? Forewarned is forearmed and maybe forewarned will get you out of your easy chair and onto the floor for the exercises that will make you fitter and the baby's chances better.

The incidence of cesarean delivery, once the rare procedure resorted to only in extreme circumstances, has risen from 5 percent in 1968 to 13 percent today. In some hospitals it runs as high as 30 percent, and it is expected that the national average will go as high as 25 percent in the next few years. One baby in four! Cesareans are not safe. No major surgery is. Cesareans are not a painless way to have a baby. The "normal" mother having a "normal" baby in the "normal" way will be giving and taking nourishment in minutes after the baby arrives. The cesarean mother and baby don't even get to love each other.

And then there are forceps. If you arrive at delivery tired, weak, tense, and loaded with trigger points (backache sufferers are loaded with trigger points), delivery pain is about to be compounded by referred pain. If you are not up to the job or are in screaming agony from back pain triggered by contractions, you will be "helped." What else can they do? Besides, the number of American women needing help makes it look to the hospital people that it's a normal need. It isn't. Help may come in the form of analgesic and anesthetic agents, and every last one of them affects the baby's environment.

So suppose you are weak and full of pain, and suppose you get "help" in the form of anesthetics. You now have a slow down in the labor process. Someone says "push" from far off and the miserable effort that ensues couldn't push a baby out of a wet paper bag. "Push, mother. Push, now," keeps echoing from somewhere, but you wish everyone would go out to the movies and let you sleep.

Obviously someone has to get that baby out, and here come the forceps. Now the way is paved for future headaches, facial pain, tinnitis, stiff neck and shoulder syndromes, TMJD, and misery. Why? Because physically unfit young mothers come to marriage and birthing with no knowledge of themselves or what they need to face the normal emergency called labor. Because birth moved from the bed to the operating table in a hospital where instruments and drugs are "normal." Because we haven't realized who pays the price in future aches and pains— Little Who-sis.

Improving the Picture for Yourself

The exercise section which follows will provide you with the special work you need to prepare yourself. The myotherapy in preparation for labor can also be used in the labor room, especially if there is back pain.

If you have always been either an athlete or a dancer, things look good for all three of you. There isn't a reason in the world why you shouldn't keep on skiing, hiking, riding, swimming, playing tennis or enjoying any of the other delightful ways you play. Obstetricians and sports physiologists generally agree that women can and should continue in sports as long as they feel comfortable. One of our students, a tiny person having her first baby, ran in the Boston Marathon the day before the baby chose to arrive.

141

This for those who have maiden aunts around who need reassurance: the danger to the fetus during the mother's physical activity is minimal. The uterus itself is extremely protective. The fetus is further protected as it floats in its bag of water (amniotic fluid). Like an egg in a sealed jar, it cannot be injured when shaken.

While the ligaments in the pelvic area have to support the additional and constantly growing weight of pregnancy and could be susceptible to stretching and tearing, normal activities without emotional stress are not harmful. I added that note about emotional stress because if there is emotional stress connected with the coming birth, there may also be trigger points waiting to fire. Athletes and dancers always have a few trigger points around. If that is the case, know that you are at double risk already, under stress and housing trigger points. Don't overdo or overstrain and unlock the triggering mechanism. If it happens anyway, check the section on sports injuries in Chapter 7 (Athletes, Weekend Sportsmen, and Their Pains).

During pregnancy institute a weekly search for trigger points in the buttocks, groin, legs, and lower back, not only as a protection for sports but in readiness for a sudden game you might have to play with no rain check.

The experts claim that pregnancy causes water retention in some and those people will be susceptible to strains and sprains. I would agree, but if you start swelling don't sit down and put on fat—look to your diet, and take the trigger points out of the offending limbs.

It is suggested by some that elastic stockings be worn whenever possible. It's hard to know exactly why. Elastic stockings are a crutch that no healthy person should don and sick people aren't up to. They will not eliminate the spasm causing swollen veins and joints. Get rid of the trigger points, do the exercises, and go play.

SPORTS DURING PREGNANCY

Being able to enjoy sports during pregnancy (or any other time) is the payoff for doing some important preparation in the form of exercise. The word exercise, once considered beneath contempt, is now very much in vogue. The meaning of the word, however, is imprecise. Which exercises? In what order? For how long? Where? When? With whom? Most of those questions can be answered, "Any way you enjoy." Which exercises and in what order, however, need explanation and at least for a while, direction.

First you use warm-ups. They lead off the exercise section, Your Basic Fitness Program to Keep Pain Away, in Chapter 10. If you precede your game or sport with three to five minutes of warm-up exercises, your muscles will be 20 percent more efficient, which means better performance and a better score. It also means less chance of injuring a muscle.

Stretching exercises are done after the body is thoroughly warm and feels both loose and supple. *Never* begin a session with stretches, jumping jacks, skips, or running. A daily routine of stretching exercises (see the following section, Exercises to Do During Pregnancy) after warm-up, of course, will keep muscles flexible and at full resting length. These exercises are a must, especially if your sport is of the quick-stop-and-start variety such as basketball or racquet games. This program will improve your skill immensely if you continue it as a pregame program after the baby is born.

If you are a golfer the experts suggest that pregnancy may cause back pain. Certainly it can, but so can your mother-in-law. To guard against any "pulled" muscles, which are really muscles in spasm due to trigger points, chase down the slightest pain with someone's elbow and do your stretch and golf exercises.

Horseback riding? Why not? Think of the egg in the sealed jar. The only danger would be a sudden stop if you were thrown, so pick your mount carefully.

Skiing is pretty hard on beginners, more exhausting than dangerous since a beginner spends most of the day climbing out of sitzmarks. But there's no reason why the expert shouldn't ski. I did some of my best racing in February. The baby came in May. Unless she is going for broke, the expert rarely falls. Cross country skiing would be ideal. You get the workout, it costs little or nothing, and you avoid the long wait in lift lines at downhill areas.

Water skiing is not recommended by the experts, and here I agree. If you go slow it's a drag and hard work. If you go fast you might get water in the birth canal, and the water close to shore, where water skiing is done, is polluted.

143

Fencing isn't worth the risk of a punctured uterus.

I was amazed to read that the "experts" even included skydiving in their deliberations. Naturally, they said it was not on the recommended list, too much of a jolt, but the fact that someone had the temerity to bring it up means that we are making progress.

Athletic women have many advantages over sedentary women. They have less fatigue, swelling, back pain, and depression. Their muscles are in excellent condition so they have faster, easier deliveries. One study made of 729 female athletes showed that 87 percent had faster deliveries than nonathletes and the time spent in the second stage of labor was half the norm. Figures were the same for both top and mediocre athletes, suggesting that overall conditioning and not skill or strength is the determining factor.

There are other advantages to being active, and for a wonder they accrue to the person most sinned against most of the time, Little Who-sis. Exercise improves both the physiological response and the circulation which is vital to the baby's growth, and it ensures good muscle tone. It is this last which shortens time and facilitates the birth.

The experts checked up on athletic performance after childbirth and found that many athletes turned in better performances than before carrying and delivering a child. And to be sure not one of them ever wrote me the kind of letter I get regularly since appearing on "Today." "Dear Miss Prudden: I've had four children in as many years and gained twenty pounds with each one. What shall I do now?!"

Here's what you do now. Exercise—

EXERCISES TO DO DURING PREGNANCY

Open Knee Bend

You will need strong legs as you grow heavier, and you don't want to get fat thighs, so do knee bends. The open knee bend will help too with crotch flexibility.

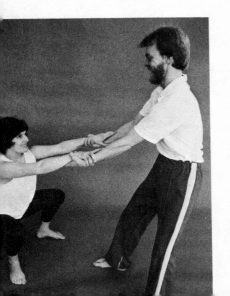

Start with feet a little apart and turned out slightly. Go down into a deep knee bend with arms extended in front and feet flat on the floor. It you have trouble keeping the heels down, enlist someone's help. Have her or him face you while you hold hands. Start with three and work up to ten. Do them every time you use the bathroom. This will keep you doing them most of the day.

Crotch Stretch

Sit with feet drawn up, sole to sole, close to your body. Grasp your ankles and rest your elbows on your thighs. Press down on the thighs with your elbows with gentle, bouncing pressure while your partner applies more weight to your knees. Close your eyes and try to find out where the muscles are resisting. If you want to see how well this concentration works, have some-one hold a ruler by your knee while you press down without concentrating, with the eyes open. Then close your eyes and think away that tight spot. The ruler will show that the knees have dropped still further. Do the gentle bounces for at least ten seconds and then release. If you let go suddenly you will experience discomfort. Relax and repeat twice more.

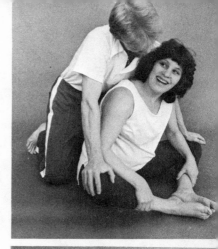

Low Back Stretch

Sitting with feet placed sole to sole and drawn up close to the body, grasp the ankles and with the help of your partner, try to move your head down to touch your feet in gentle bounces. Use the same eyes-closed concentration as for the previous exercise to find the tight places and release them. Have someone watch your lower back, even if you are so flexible that you can touch your feet with your head. He will see the muscles give up tension and stretch even further. Do those bounces for at least ten seconds. Relax and repeat twice more

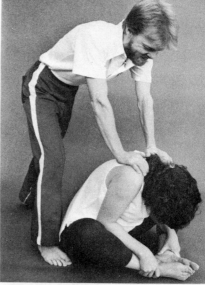

Low Back and Hamstring Stretch

Take the spread-leg position while seated on the floor and lean straight forward, keeping knees stiff and turning feet slightly out. Have the partner press down on the shoulders in eight easy bounces. As you are stretched try to concentrate on the tight spots and let them go. After eight bounces, sit straight for a second or two and repeat. Do four.

The exercises for stretch employing another person's help will get faster results than those in which each person must do his or her own pulling. That is because the whole body can relax while someone else does the work.

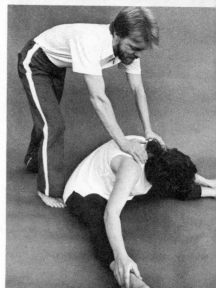

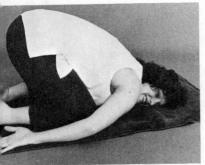

PRE- AND POSTNATAL RELAXATION TECHNIQUES

Knee-Chest Rest

To relieve pressure from the growing child inside you, kneel on slightly spread knees. Put one ear on floor and bring both arms to rest on floor alongside the legs. Rest for one minute like this, then change the head so that the other ear rests on floor. Two minutes gives your back some stretch and rests your pelvic area.

Prone Rest—One Pillow

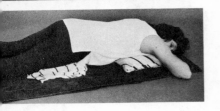

A tired back rests best with one knee bent whether you are prone or supine. The pillow under the knee changes the angle of the pelvis and takes further strain off the back. It also makes room for expanding tummy.

Prone Rest—Two Pillows

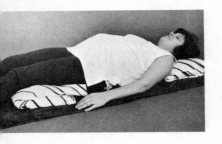

For those who have rested prone all their lives, the sudden appearance of a bulge in front can be distressing. If you want to lie face down, put a pillow above and below your bulge, and go ahead.

Supine Rest

Circulation is often slowed because of the weight of the child against the large veins coming up into the pelvis. So when you rest on your back, put a pillow under your knees. With elevated legs, circulation will increase, which will make you less tired and your feet and ankles less swollen, and will help prevent varicose veins.

WHY YOUR BABY NEEDS MYOTHERAPY

When I first started taking babies on TV to demonstrate "baby exercise," I discovered that some of them did not like to have their clothes taken off, even though studio lights are more than warm enough. Comfortable, happy babies do like to get rid of their clothes. Then I thought "Uh-oh, Mom probably keeps the kid in cotton wool and the nursery is really an incubator." Now I wonder if a change in temperature hitting spasmed muscles could have something to do with it.

My own first baby was born into a dreary climate and screamed for three months. Her grandmother ran the roost, and me. The baby was not to be picked up. The baby was to be fed on time, not later than every four hours, but not any sooner either. Poor little baby, poor ignorant young mother. Even today the one person in the world most likely to have a baby one day, the high school girl, while told where babies come from and how to get one or not get one, is taught nothing about what to do with one once it gets here.

Today I would go over every inch of that little body looking for the trigger points that were causing the spasm that was causing the pain that was causing the screaming that was causing the colic as air was swallowed hour after excruciating hour. The sad thing about discovering a way to ease pain is finding it too late to help your own. For my own children I am too late, but let's do what we can for yours, and for those yet to come.

Being Born: A Painful Chore

Being born is rather like riding a sled down a steep, icy hill into traffic at a cross street. If one thing doesn't hit you something else will.

Sometimes one runs into trouble even before starting down that hill. The meals served in the rooming house where the baby is putting itself together may be less than nutritious. Perhaps the cocktail hour has a way of running into the dinner hour—or even replacing the dinner hour. Maybe the lady who runs the rooming house lives in a stress-filled atmosphere that loads up everybody's system with adrenaline. Or possibly she takes something to stop the adrenaline, like a tranquilizer or three.

The baby may not have chosen to be born, but then, the woman may not have chosen to have the baby. Things could be rough all around. Everybody talks about the Nirvana of the Womb—how peaceful it is in there, far from strife and the eleven o'clock news. Who says? For a long time we thought babies didn't hear, see, or feel anything and that smiles were really gas pains. "Circumcision is nothing; why he doesn't feel a thing." Where is the proof? Regression through hypnosis says otherwise.

147

We don't know but what it might be very different indeed. Remember when Alice started to grow and the room got smaller and smaller? The same thing happens to babies. That of course is normal, though I imagine it could become uncomfortable. But uncomfortable is hardly the word for what happens if the baby is tipped over a little so that its head is on its shoulder or the shoulder shoved up toward its ear. With less and less room it might have to hold that position for quite a while.

THE BABY WHO ARRIVED IN A HURRY

If the womb is Nirvana, what a descent into the pits birth must be. Mike was born in two and a half hours, and his head was so battered that three weeks later his eyes were still bloodshot. He seemed to recover, however, and in a few months he was a bright little wiggler who loved to roll around on the floor getting into and out of corners almost as fast as his three-year-old sister. Suddenly all that changed.

Mike began to scream. He screamed day and night. He stopped only when utterly exhausted. Before his also exhausted mother could get to sleep, he was screaming again.

He gave up wiggling. The light of curiosity went out of him and he never smiled at all, just screamed. Nerves were so frazzled that the place got to be a madhouse with everyone jumpy, including the nurse who came in days to take care of him while his mother went to work. No way to live.

I had seen this before in children who had "superficial birth injuries." All his mother could tell me was that he had arrived looking like a war casualty. Well, what does superficial mean? In the medical dictionary the word means "pertaining to or near the surface." Ask yourself, where are the muscles covering the head and face—they are very near the surface. If accidents lay trigger points in the muscles at the site of insult, Mike must have had many. We had only 15 minutes during a workshop in North Carolina to explain to Mike's mother the theory of trigger points and myotherapy.

Mike wasn't screaming when she brought him, but the minute I put very gentle pressure on the frontalis muscle in the front of his head, he howled. Remembering that his eyes had been swollen shut after that tumultuous arrival, I circled the muscles around his eyesockets (orbicularis oculi). The howling increased to a roar. I stopped pressing and he stopped howling.

"I think it's trigger points. There is no guarantee that it will work," I told her. She wanted to try. I showed her how to search for and erase the trigger points. Check with Chapter 5, on head and face pain, and you can see what she had to do, little by little, day by day.

We left North Carolina right after the workshop, but there was no such escape for Mike's mother. She knew what she was in for. She waited in the parking lot until all the cars had departed, then holding the little fellow in her lap, she began by just touching the places we had told her were harboring the trigger points that caused Mike's pain. She wasn't disappointed, the screaming began. After clearing the trigger points she picked him up to "get rid of the gas," the air he swallowed while screaming. He grabbed for her hair (his security blanket), and she felt his taut little body relax. A few minutes later he was asleep and she put him in the car seat and drove home.

That night Mike seemed to his father to be brighter, and he even played a little. During the night, when he cried, his mother again touched the trigger points around his face and he went off to sleep. Nobody who has not held a screaming, jerking little baby whose arms slash every which way and whose head bangs from side to side can know what a relief it is to feel that baby relax and then sleep.

Next day the nurse said Mike was more like his old self, but when his mother began to nurse him he started to scream again. If you will look at the drawing of the face muscles (Plate 12 in Appendix 1), you will notice the masseter muscle in the jaw. That muscle contracts when the baby nurses, and that muscle of Mike's had turned the very pleasant business of feeding into a nightmare for him.

Mike's mother just worked on the little face, and the screaming stopped. He went back to nursing and then to sleep. The nurse, who had taken care of that poor little yeller for months, was astounded. "What did you do?" When it was explained, the nurse who had many years of experience with babies, said simply, "Teach me."

Within weeks, Mike had stopped screaming except when his trigger points were pressed, and by then they were being pressed, not just touched.

He was back to playing and wiggling, starting an honest-to-goodness crawl, and would even stand if someone offered a hand. The worst was over. No, the worst had been avoided.

THE BABY WHO COULDN'T STAND UP

Alyssa had trouble at the other extremity—her legs. She was a happy, loving baby who slept well, and played sweetly with her fingers and her daddy's nose. But she wouldn't stand up. Long after the "should books" said she should be standing and bouncing her little body on gently bending knees, Alyssa was still sitting. Not only would she not stand up in her playpen as most babies did at her age, she wouldn't stay on her feet when her mother tried to stand her up in her lap. While Mike screamed most of the time, Alyssa screamed only when stood up. While Mike cried for hours on end; Alyssa stopped her wails the second she was allowed to sit or lie down.

Pain that is called teething can go on for months, and, while it drives everyone up a wall, parents don't become frightened unless it continues after the appearance of the teeth. Pain that goes with standing is usually something that demands medical attention at once. Alyssa had her first X-rays before she was a year old. She was checked for fractures and hip dislocation and congenital anomalies. Everything was "normal," and her mother was told to wait awhile; it was probably just growing pains.

The parents waited awhile. Alyssa still couldn't stand or walk like her playmates. They decided it was time to see a specialist and settled on an orthopedist. He eventually called in a neurologist. It was decided that Alyssa should be fitted for braces.

As it happens, that was the week we held our first pain erasure clinic. I was working in the teacher's lounge with a cardiologist who had severe contractures after brain surgery, when Ally was plunked down on the table. She was cheerful as her mother explained the trouble. Well, if trigger points were the villain, it wouldn't take long to find out. I looked at the sweet little face as I pressed against the adductor muscle on one tiny thigh. The little face screwed into a mask of baby misery. By the

150

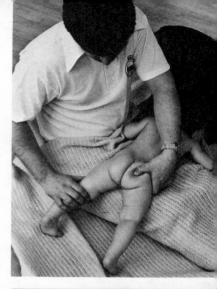

time I reached the muscle just above the knee she was sobbing, so I stopped. Alyssa stopped crying. I started hunting again, this time in the lower leg, and the baby cried the whole way down. When I stopped, she stopped. There wasn't time to do more. but there is always time later with babies.

I showed the mother what to do and gave her a "map" of the legs marked where I thought she would find the tender spots. In two weeks Ally was standing without any pain and, shortly after that, walking like any normal baby. Today she has straight, strong, beautiful legs, and her mother says she never walks, she just runs and runs.

When you have seen your doctor to confirm that there is no sign of disease, don't think braces. Babies hate braces, and braces cause their own trigger points. Rather, think trigger points and spasm. It's easy enough to find out. Simply press muscles in the problem area.

It isn't always Mother anymore who has charge of the baby and its problems. Ron brought Kim to us after three months in appliances designed to force little feet to turn out. They hadn't. Ron wanted to know if myotherapy would help. I told him about Alyssa and we started.

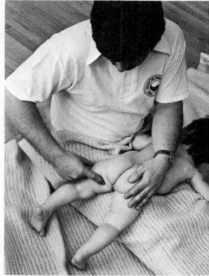

TRIGGER POINT ERASURE IN BABIES

The first place to look for trouble is, as usual, in the gluteals, the seat. Check with spots 1, 2, and 3 on Plate 5 in Appendix 1. Using the thumb instead of the elbow, press for about five seconds. Don't be surprised at the protest that greets your first endeavors. The trigger points will soon be gone and there will be no more tears. After pressing one or two spots on each side, do the knee-bending exercises described under Hamstring Stretch, later in this chapter.

Next, the adductors. Go right down the inside of the thigh at half-inch intervals pressing with your thumb or finger. Start in spot 36, shown on Plate 8. Repeat the knee-bending exercises and do the hamstring stretch as well (see page 157).

The lower leg too needs to be searched. Start at spot 47, the top of the soleus (shown on Plate 8), and go down the inner aspect of the back of the leg. Follow with the inside of the leg.

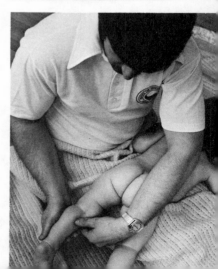

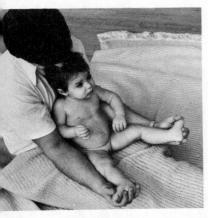

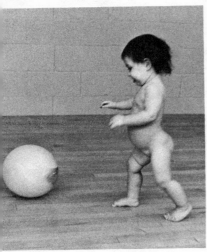

The stretch for a foot that turns in is done by helping the entire leg to turn out. It is assumed that a baby who has been put into braces for feet that turn in has been X-rayed for perthes, a congenital condition of the hips, and that the X-rays are negative.

Hold the baby on your lap and turn the little legs out to rhythm. Turn on music and exercise to it. Babies love rhythm, music, love, holding, attention—and you. Do the leg stretch dozens of times a day.

The improvement in Kim was marked. But more things happened to Kim than a change in the direction of her feet. Because of the exercise, her whole body is slim, strong, and coordinated. She has strong ties to her parents who work with her. As a result of the massage, her body is remarkably relaxed. And all these qualities together make for a healthy, happy baby whose sports future is already assured.

THE VALUE OF EXERCISES WITH BABY

Once in the world, babies should be encouraged to stretch cramped muscles and contract those that have done most of their growing in a constant state of overstretch. A study of an infant's muscles will suggest to you that many of the major posture problems of children, and grown-ups as well, started in the womb: the soft abdominal area that shows up later as a potbelly; the contracted pectoral muscles and overstretched back muscles that contribute to being round shouldered; even the shortened hamstrings that can lead to backache. You cannot begin too soon to counteract the effects of cramped quarters.

As we already know, Americans are not very disciplined when it comes to exercise, but if we begin soon enough and are consistent long enough, we can help establish in our babies the habit of exercising. What is needed is a pattern that is adhered to without deviation, that is, to exercise the baby at the same time, in the same place, and with the same aids every single day. We like to begin the following exercise program as soon after birth as a few days.

The Place

The floor is the best place for baby exercises for several reasons. It provides good support, it puts the mother on the same level with her baby; and it provides a feeling of space. The baby's first days and nights are bound to be spent in confined quarters. Bassinets, cribs, prams, and arms offer security and warmth, but not a wide horizon. Then, too, there is always the hope that the mother who exercises her baby is herself down on the floor where exercise is easily done, and will begin a program of her own.

Aids

A big towel makes almost any floor space acceptable. If the room is drafty, an infrared bulb in a gooselnecked lamp is ideal. First, it will keep the baby warm in almost any weather. Also, you can easily determine how much heat the baby is getting because it will shine on the back of your neck first.

You will need a clock. Too much exercise on Monday leads to none on Tuesday. Limit your time to five minutes a session at first, and if there is a good record player handy, both you and the baby will enjoy timing movement to a good beat. Two bands of any pop record will do the job, but if you did your own prenatal exercises every day to the same music, use it now, too. The baby heard and remembers.

The Time

It really makes very little difference what time of day you exercise your baby. There are advantages, however, in conducting your "classes" on a regular schedule and at those times of day when you would ordinarily be changing the baby's clothes or giving it a bath. This will eliminate unnecessary dressing and undressing. It should also be done when there is no chance of interruption, so take the phone off the hook.

Whenever there is a diaper change, do a little of each exercise so that the baby's body is constantly directed into the full range of correct movement. This constant reinforcement of good movement patterns will be "remembered" when the baby's own proprioception is developed. (Proprioception is the reception of stimuli within muscles and tendons; it determines how we handle ourselves in space.)

153

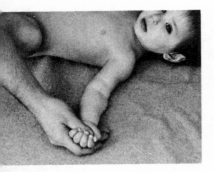

THE EXERCISES

Arm Stretches

When you are ready to start, undress your baby and put it down on the floor. Do not separate its body from yours as you place it on the exercise towel, but lean down with it. Only when its back is in contact with the floor do you take away that safe feeling of being a part of you.

A baby has a natural self-supporting grip when it is born, and if you help, it need never be lost. Strong hands are a plus even for babies. Let the baby grasp your thumbs, and close your fingers over its hands so that the grip is maintained. As you put pressure on its arms you will find your thumbs grasped more tightly. This reflex may be a holdover from some remote age when an ancestor needed it for survival. Like the swimming reflex you will read about shortly, it comes with the baby, and stays with the baby as long as it is used.

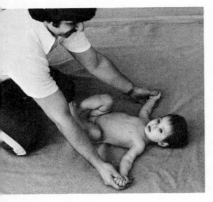

Chest and Back Stretch

Pull the little arms gently and slowly at first to a full lateral stretch. In the beginning there will be some resistance. Its little computer hasn't been programmed for such action as yet. For a long time it will be harder for your baby to give up tension in its muscles and relax them, than it will to contract them. (This is also true of adults.) Unless they are taught to consciously relax their muscles, they suffer from many aches and pains, notably in the neck, shoulders, head, and back. Now with myotherapy that tendency should be reversed.

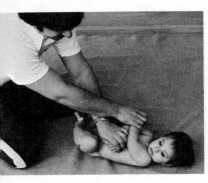

When a baby resists stretch, it is working against resistance, as though your hands were barbells. It is building strength. When the arms stretch easily and long, flexibility is being developed. Either way you win.

Next, draw the little arms across the chest. This movement stretches the back and exercises the shoulders as no random movement can.

And talk to your baby. Your voice is new now, but soon it will be the pivot of the baby's world. Give your baby the gift of your voice every chance you get, and remember, it is the tone that is heard. Sing, too, sing anything, in tune or out, lyrics don't matter. Words like *one, two, three, four* may be just numbers to you, but to your baby they mean, "Here I am, here you are, here we are together, and I love you."

Do about eight arm stretches. Don't hurry, it's the complete all-the-way-out-and-all-the-way-in movement you are after. Set up a rhythm as soon as you can. Babies already understand rhythm. Remember your heartbeat all those months and the baby's heart beating twice as fast.

Overhead Stretch

Next, draw the baby's arms up overhead and then back down to the sides. Every time the arms reach upward the little chest expands to make room for more oxygen. More oxygen means more fuel to both body and mind. Also, using the lungs will make them grow more efficient. In addition, the shoulder joints are being introduced to a new angle. One it would not be able to attain for itself for a long, long time. Do eight stretches.

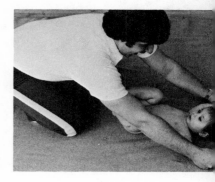

Shoulder Rotations

Hold the baby's arm above the wrist. Gently rotate inward until the palm is on the floor. Then rotate outward until the palm faces up. Do six on each side to slow music. Then do them both at the same time. At first little babies do not make many movements involving one limb and not the other. Alternating one arm up and the other arm down is a very advanced motion indeed.

But you have a very advanced baby. Did you know that if you spoke to your baby in one language, your spouse in another, and big sister in a third, by the time she had learned to talk she would speak in all three? Human beings use only about one tenth of their brain, and the rest seems to lie fallow. Could that be because we don't develop more of it when we are just starting out?

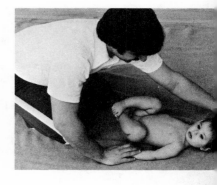

Leg Stretches

Your baby's knees have been bent for months. Imagine how you would feel cramped into the back seat of a Volkswagen and forced to ride there for six or seven hours at a time. Your first thought would be, "When can I get out of here and stretch my legs?" The baby likes leg stretches, too. Grasp the ankles and pull gently out, then push as gently back in. Do about eight.

155

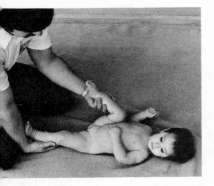

The Bicycle

The "bicycle" does the stretching that helps strengthen legs. The alternation of the legs, as one is stretched and the other pushed to the knee-bent position, counteracts the natural contraction tendency, making an extension of the leg easier and more complete. Furthermore, it is a real lifesaver because babies love it. Use this exercise to help you over rough spots in the doctor's office, in an airplane, when the baby is tired of lying in its crib, and also just for fun.

The Inchworm

No mother who has waited through those last two months of pregnancy is really surprised to see her baby push itself up into the corner of a crib or even halfway across the room. There are several times during that waiting period when Little Who-sis got both legs together and almost pushed her dinner back up. The only thing preventing most babies from practicing this activity is lack of leg room.

When you place the baby in the prone position its legs will probably curl up under the body. Place your thumbs against the soles of its feet and hold fast. There will be a mighty shove and the tiny body will move forward. Those legs are strong; see that they stay that way. Imagine trying to inch your own body across a rough surface with just leg power. See what I mean? We are born strong and then allow ourselves to deteriorate. Pound for pound your baby could give you a good race. Try for two pushes at first and add whatever the baby wants to manage. The other exercises described are passive ones, meaning you do most of the work. But pushing across the floor is entirely the baby's decision and the baby does the work. Later you will be able to encourage all kinds of floor progression by placing shiny articles a little ahead.

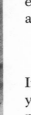

The Back Arch

Imagine how you would feel if some ill fate made it necessary for you to spend a night curled up in a child's crib. Long before morning you would be praying for a chance to straighten your back. The baby's back has been rounded for months. It likes new

positions. So pick up the spindly legs and arch the back a little.

Hold that position for a slow count of three while making appropriate noises that would go with such an adventure. For the baby it is an adventure. It probably would be for you too if two enormous hands picked up your legs and arched your back! Kim has reached the "wheelbarrow stage," when the baby can push up to look around.

Hamstring Stretch

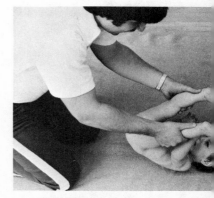

With your thumbs against the baby's calves and your fingers over the knees, carefully straighten the legs. As you bring the feet toward the head, lift the seat from the floor. It is not necessary to go very far at first. The baby, like many adults who have spent too much time sitting, will not find this exercise easy. After you have done the stretch once, let the baby kick free for a few seconds. Then you repeat it. Do three or four.

The last two exercises, like the hamstring stretch, are for stretch. Incidentally, the exercises are useful for anyone whose feet turn in, babies, older children and grown-ups alike.

In the first of these, as you hold the thighs open, bend both knees and then stretch the legs to the straight-legged wide-spread position. Do four.

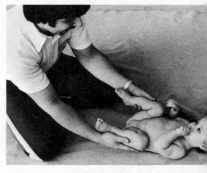

The second is to bring the baby's feet close to the buttocks and press the knees open. Hold open for a slow count of three, relax and repeat. Do four.

Babyhood is when the fastest growth and changes are taking place. You are in on the beginning when everything counts more than it ever will again.

SEEKING MASSAGE FOR BABIES

Remember Mike who screamed all the time, and Alyssa who wouldn't stand? It wasn't until Mike's screams had continued for months that he was found to have muscle trouble. Alyssa's muscles weren't suspected until she passed the walking stage and was still sitting. What a waste of time. We should know our babies' bodies like the back of our own hands. Seeking massage offers real help as you search for sensitive muscles.

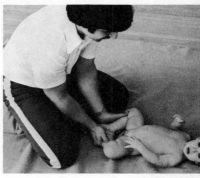

We first came across baby massage in a book by Dr. Frederick LeBoyer, *Loving Hands*. He had spent time in the East

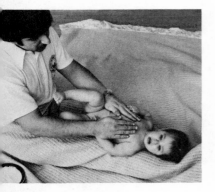

and had studied women working with their babies. (It was also Dr. LeBoyer who wrote *Birth Without Violence*, an absolute must for anyone planning a baby. There are now hospitals in America using the LeBoyer system in which babies are considered to be travel-weary people who should be welcomed quietly and gently without bright lights, noise, and rude temperature transitions.)

What is needed? A warm room, a large and a small towel, and a bowl of warm oil—coconut, olive, or almond.

The massager sits on the floor, the baby lies on its back on the massager's knees. The warm oil is first spread on your hands and then transferred to the area being massaged.

Chest

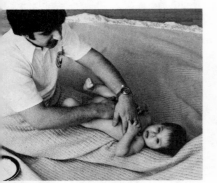

Lay both hands on the chest and move them outward to both sides, around, and back to the center. Follow the outline of the baby's ribs, both hands at the same time, as if smoothing open the pages of a book. Do this three or four times.

Then place your right hand on the baby's right side (between the hip and the rib cage) and move it across the abdomen and chest to the left shoulder. As it ends its move start the left hand at the left side and move across to the right shoulder. One hand follows the other in a steady rhythm. Do several.

Arms

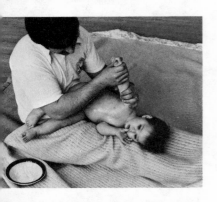

Turn the baby onto its left side with its body close to yours. Take the baby's right hand in your right hand and place your left hand around the arm and shoulder. Gently squeeze the limb in a milking action to the wrist. As you reach the wrist, grasp the hand and wrist in your left hand and repeat the squeezing action with your right hand. Repeat on the other side only after doing the next exercise on this side.

Towel Wring

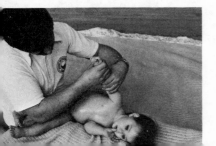
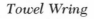

Both your hands start at the baby's shoulder. With the gentlest of twisting motions, as though you were wringing a towel, move down the arm to the wrist. Linger awhile at the wrist and then repeat.

Now do both this exercise and the one before with the other arm.

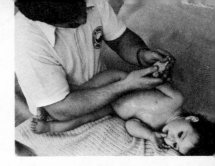

Hands

Hold the baby's wrist with both hands, one over the other. Work your thumbs one after the other toward the fingers, massaging the palm. Uncurl the fingers over and over again.

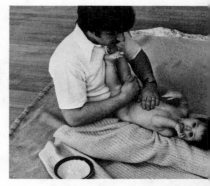

Abdomen

Bring the child closer with its legs spread. Lay your right hand at the base of the rib cage and slide the hand down toward the groin. As your hand reaches the groin, lay the left hand at the base of the rib cage and repeat. The move is made as though you were trying to empty the stomach.

After six downward strokes, grasp the child's feet in your right hand and lay your left forearm across the lower part of the abdomen. Using the forearm as an anchor, stretch the baby's legs straight up to further relax the abdomen. This allows the massage to penetrate deeper. Repeat the stroking as before.

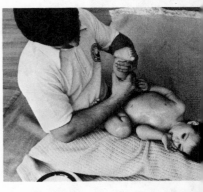

Legs

Slide the baby farther down your legs so that its buttocks are over your thighs. Use the same exercise as for the arms, gently squeezing up toward the raised foot. Remember to spend extra time at the ankles as when doing the towel wring.

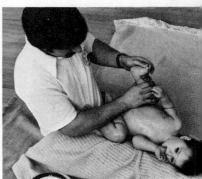

Foot

The foot is treated the same way as the hands. Grasp one foot in both hands and work your thumbs along the child's sole. Then use your palm to stretch the heel cords.

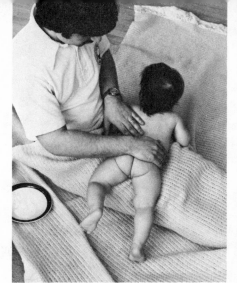 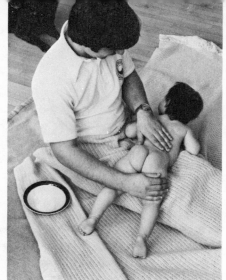

Back

This is the most important of all. Never skip this. Place the baby face down across your thighs, its head to the left side. Then proceed:

Across the back. Seesaw your hand across the back, starting at the neck and working down over the buttocks, then back up again.

Down the back. The right hand holds the buttocks firm by pressing against the backs of the thighs. The left hand starts on the shoulders, touching the neck, and moves slowly, with no break in the rhythm, downward along the spine and over the buttocks.

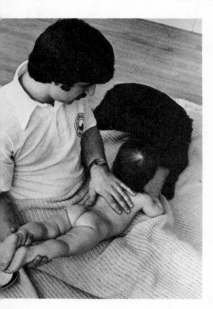

From Shoulders to Heels

Grasp the ankles with the right hand and stretch the baby full length. The heels should be a little higher than the head. Slide your left hand all the way down from shoulders to heels in one steady movement.

Face, Forehead

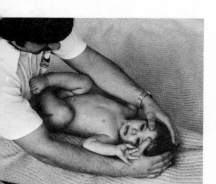

The baby should be returned to its back, legs spread or curled, and torso close to you. Place the fingers of both hands in the middle of its forehead. The tips of your fingers move sideways along the eyebrows several times.

Bridge of the nose. Place both hands on the baby's face and move the thumbs upward toward the forehead along the sides of the baby's nose.

Down along the nose. Apply the thumbs lightly to the baby's closed eyelids. Move down and slightly sideways to the corners of the mouth. Gently stretch the mouth outward and return your thumbs to baby's forehead.

Ideally one begins this exercise and massage while the baby is still almost newborn. To these should be added getting the baby into warm water with the mother or father. The bathtub is a good place to start. The baby has a reflex that prevents inhaling while the face (the whole face) is underwater. The baby also has reflex swimming motions, and both are in effect for four months. After that the reflexes (babies are swimmers before they are walkers) begin to wane. Get my book *Your Baby Can Swim* (see the Sources section for details), and add it to the treasures you are providing your baby.

MASSAGE AND MYOTHERAPY FOR PREVENTION

When I first started using myotherapy on babies I suggested to the mothers that they follow the trigger point work with a gentle massage à la LeBoyer. But once, while I was demonstrating it, one of the babies began to cry loudly. I ran my finger down the inside of the thigh, the place where Alyssa's trigger points had nested. Howl! I rubbed gently near the knee. No howl. Up two inches. Howl! We had found a trigger point. Then we noticed for the first time that one foot was turned in. No one had noticed this condition until pain called it to our attention. Out with the trigger point. Three days later, no howls.

If, after the oil is applied for massage, you press along the lines shown on the illustrations of the limbs in Appendix 1, your chances are good of finding hidden trigger points that could cause trouble later—trouble such as growing pains, turned in or turned out feet, or a round back. If as you run your fingers with some little pressure along either side of the spine you elicit discomfort, you may well have found the trigger points that later

161

could cause back problems. Such back problems could include scoliosis, or spinal curvature. Most cases of scoliosis do not surface before about age eleven, but one little boy of four was sent to us to prepare him with flexibility exercises for his operation. He never had the operation.

Don't wait until you have a problem. Seeking massage searches out trouble in a muscle that is sensitive; myotherapy corrects the condition and prevents complications.

Erase the Pains of Aging or Hurting

Older people do have more pain than young people, but not because of age. They have more pain because they have had more time in which to lay down the causes of pain. The major cause is not age per se. The same pain in a young or even middle-aged person would be the signal for immediate investigation—something must be wrong. But we have convinced ourselves that pain is something that just happens to old people. "After all, what do you expect at your age?"

And the old person has had more "help" for his or her pain. First, in the form of bed rest, which is almost standard. Then there are crutches, canes, braces, corsets, traction, and mind-jumbling tranquilizers. Most people can handle age. What they can't handle is constant, unremitting pain, along with most of the methods used to relieve it. Fortunately, now we have myotherapy.

WE CAN COUNTERACT DETERIORATION

As we age, we don't have to deteriorate at the average and expected rate. We can plan our lives so that we will be safe behind the impregnable walls provided by strength, health, and independence. That, however, calls for vigilance and hard work. Through exercise and good nutrition, and with the help of myotherapy, we can and must stay healthy.

We must also guard against agoraphobia, which is the fear of open spaces or any place outside the house. It often assures isolation. This is followed as a rule by a deterioration of mental

163

faculties often called senility. Actually we see the same thing in deprived children. They appear to be dull. They appear to lack the ability to react positively. The wise older warrior plans against such an invader by going forth into the world on regular forays. He or she keeps the mind occupied with books. (Today's older person at least knows how to read!)

And let's remember that many of our mentally active scientists, artists, authors, composers, musicians, and statesmen have done their best work in later life.

Sleep, too, is often a problem for the older person. It will come more easily to the physically active person. He will be more relaxed, sleep more readily and more soundly. Pain, which can ruin sleep, can be taken care of with myotherapy. And if all else fails, what's wrong with a nice warm bed and a good light for reading? If you can't sleep, don't fret. Read. People really don't need as much sleep as they think they do.

Enjoy the Active Life

For those who want to stay in shape or get into shape there is the whole out-of-doors. An excellent book by Ralph H. Hopp, *Enjoying the Active Life After Fifty*, gives a wealth of information. See the Sources section for detail.

There are many ways to enjoy the outdoor world without going so far as to take up jogging—walking, for example. I don't mean down the street to the supermarket, but over the hills and far away. Add photography to walking, and you have both motivation and something to show for your efforts later on. Bird-watching is another good diversion. It calls for being where the birds are, and since where birds are you will also find bird-watchers, you may widen your circle of friends as well as your knowledge.

Camping can be enjoyed by folks over 65. Just remember that the first two nights on the ground may be a bit uncomfortable. After that, it's easy, and challenging.

Hunting doesn't happen to be my bag except when the shooting is done with a camera. But my father used to go hunting in Maine on his vacation. He'd leave home a nervous wreck. After two weeks, he'd return, bearded, brown, and smelling of the woods and man and snow. After that he could stand the newspaper business for another year.

Fishing—there's a sport that's always good. It can be extremely peaceful, you are almost sure to get a tan, and maybe dinner, too. There is usually some place not too far from home where you can drop a line in and even if you reel it in empty, it's a lovely way to spend a day.

Swimming is another activity that isn't denied even the most elderly.

Boating doesn't have to mean big boating. Rowboats, canoes, kayaks, even rubber rafts all contribute to the fun of just being afloat. Sailing is like having wings.

Biking is something you learned as a kid and haven't forgotten.

Tennis of course is "in" today, but then it was "in" when today's oldsters were youngsters. Many learned the game then and if they stay in shape, they can play and enjoy the game still. My mother-in-law at 50 consistently creamed me when I was 25. She didn't even get winded because she kept me running all around the court and I could never move her around.

Golf is traditionally the game delegated to the older generation. For years, when anyone asked me if I played golf, I said "No, not yet. When I get old I'll take it up," and I probably will.

Horseback riding is a lovely way to go—anywhere from Central Park to the Rockies. The horse does most of the work and you get to enjoy the view. The first, second, and third trip out your legs may scream. But they did when you were 20, too. I worked on a ranch in Arizona when I was 18 and found that I would get stiff riding someone else's horse for a couple of hours. My own horse had educated my muscles in a certain way and even a short exposure to a different movement would make itself felt. So hang in there.

Skiing is another wonderful way to go, especially cross country. Downhill skiing has gotten so crowded and expensive and the lift lines so long that the pleasure has become minimal. Anybody can learn cross country skiing, and a fall is usually from a standing position into soft snow, not downhill at top speed onto a bone-cracking boiler plate!

Mr. Hopp in his book is most thorough in providing sources for just about every activity. The hardest thing about taking up a sport is the first move. He makes it easy. To Mr. Hopp's list I would add one of my favorites, skin diving, a real joy and well within the ability of any swimmer. The older person who has the means to go to the Caribbean should not limit himself to a stroll on the beach. Put on fins, mask, and snorkel and see what's going on down under.

What it comes down to then is a form of war against deterioration. You can win most of the battles if you are in shape, so get there. Do as many of the exercises in Chapter 10 as you can and then find an outdoor activity and prepare for it.

HOW TO SURVIVE A HOSPITAL

If you are like me, you have no great affection for hospitals. All the same, there are times when they can be mighty handy. By October 1978, I knew there was no way of avoiding a total replacement of my left hip. I'd been through that operation some years earlier for my right one, and it was a horror story.

On that occasion, I contracted a raging case of hepatitis from the transfusions (which I'd paid for). The hours in the recovery room were spent in screaming agony from back spasms. The painkiller Demerol, to which I am allergic, was administered, and most of me rose up in hives and edema. The I.V. needle, through which dripped whatever, slipped somehow, and instead of the stuff dripping into a vein, which can handle the situation, it went into the tissues, which can't. Soon my arm was bigger than my leg. The nurse, long past the retirement age, was addicted to limiting morphine. She would prolong the intervals between injections long past the point where the pain could be controlled. It took her all morning to give a bedbath and there was no way she could move me without using my incision as a fulcrum.

But physical discomfort was not the only misery. I had made the mistake of not telling anyone I was going to the hospital. What people don't know may not hurt *them*, but in this case it hurt *me*. I was lonely and scared to be sure, but I was worse off than merely alone. I felt at the mercy of the hospital. Hospitals, it would seem, are not for patients; they are for hospital staff. It is a very uneasy position to be in, and you must guard against it. True, you may never need the help you are about to set up for yourself, but you may never need to learn to swim either. The trouble is, you can't take the precautions necessary once you are in the water!

It should not be surprising that, when I learned hip surgery was on my agenda again, I was practically a basket case.

But, since so much of my life has changed for the positive in the last few years, I began to think that maybe it doesn't have to be like that. To start with we now have myotherapy. I reasoned that if we can help aching arms in and out of casts, if we can wipe pain from spasmed backs and shoulders and the scars of open heart surgery, why shouldn't it help a postoperative hip when muscles are sure to be in spasm from the operation if nothing else?

We began at once with two things, myotherapy to my back and both legs on a regular basis and always after extreme exertion, and thermal Aqua-Ex. I was in that hot water two half hours a day, "dancing" to rock music. As the event approached I upped that to three half hours. Those two things worked so well that I was able to conduct a three-day fitness workshop in North Carolina and go into the hospital the next day. I was strong and had fairly good range. Happily, it was a different hospital with a very different attitude toward patients.

I was concerned with the choice of the doctor, what type of hip replacement he planned for me, and who was to be the nurse. The last was settled first. My good friend Dee Winslow, who is an R.N. and a myotherapist, volunteered. She would be perfect. "Beanie" Whittaker, the associate director of the institute, said she would be there. The troops were assembling, and for sure it's troops you need. Two other myotherapists, Don Whittaker and Lori Drummond, wanted to be part of the experiment (would myotherapy help postoperatively?). I felt safer by the day. All of them wore their "blues" (blue warm-up suits with white stripes down the pants) and, except for the nurse, myotherapy patches. No one ever wanted to look dumb and ask what a myotherapist was so they were accepted as hospital staff and no one ever said, "Visiting hours are over now. . . ."

Now to the doctor. I found him! I will not give his name here lest he be expelled from the rolls as a renegade, but if you need him, write to me. The first thing I did was tell him how much and why I hate hospitals. He said he understood. Then I asked to be given myotherapy right after the operation. That was fine with him so long as it did not interfere with the suture line. From what you already know about myotherapy the suture line was far from the work area, which would be in the back and lower legs for starters, coming close to the operated site only much later after healing was complete and the sutures long gone. For the record, he did the myotherapy on my back in the

167

recovery room himself. As a result, there was no screaming agony.

Next I talked to him about medication. "I'm allergic to Demerol (he wrote that down), I can tolerate morphine, and I'm not an addict. I'd like to be the one who says when I don't need it anymore since I'll be the one who is hurting." That sounded reasonable to him and that's the way it was.

I almost lost him when I said no traction. He said there would be spasm and I said there wouldn't. He took my word for it. An interesting sidelight was provided by the physical therapist. One day she came in with a bicycle and suggested I ride for five minutes. All my training had said no bike after hip surgery, but I rode anyway and it felt good. Nobody is always right. The frame around the bed that enables the patient to lift the upper body from the bed was festooned with the kind of gadgets we use for exercise—rubber straps for stretching, pulleys, weight bags, and so on—and I'd been working with them all along. Much of what I did would have horrified the medical profession, and Dee, my nurse, got a permanent crick in her neck from looking the other way.

On the third day the doctor came in with his entourage, bent my knee, and wagged it back and forth. Then, without a trace of a smile said, "Remarkable, we must try this on humans."

On the fifth day I was given a walker and crutches. I ignored both and walked limpless to the bathroom. The doctor then insisted I use the crutches for six weeks. Oh, well, the doctor had given me my way up to now. At this point I felt I should reciprocate.

Why do you need friends in a hospital? For protection! I had done it right. I had my own carefully selected nurse who could give a painless bedbath in 15 minutes. When I needed medication it was there. Neither Beanie nor Dee left my room except for supplies and assorted meals the whole first week. Beanie stayed on 24-hour duty for the second week as well. No medication was given to me while I was out of it that they didn't know about, and once I was back in my head, none that I didn't know about. If I needed something, it was there. If something bothered me, it was gone. When I went for X-rays, it was with a bodyguard; when I wanted to exercise, my walker was held stable. The I.V. was constantly monitored and stayed in the vein. As you see, I was well protected.

So start your own Hospital Protection Group, the motto of which should be, "I'll sit with you if you'll sit with me." If someone you love has to be in a hospital, think twice before leaving him or her alone.

Incidentally, since I was so painfree and cared for this second time, I became aware of other things I had missed altogether the first time. Cards come under the heading of entertainment, so if you are sending any, get funny ones. Sentiment is nice, but laughter is healing. Plants are better than cut flowers: they go home with you. Fun is essential. As hospital gifts, I got one Easter rabbit, two Easter baskets, a Raggedy Ann, six pounds of fresh lobster, and a half gallon of bourbon. When I got home I found that two trees named Hip I and Hip II had been planted in my yard as mementos.

One or two things more. If you have to go to the hospital, take your own back-rub cream from home. The stuff they use in the hospital can give your back a terminal case of diaper rash. Take along a couple of pairs of men's pajamas, even if you are the most feminine of ladies. Elbows and backs need protection from the detergents sheets are washed in. If you are addicted to a hot-water bottle for cold feet, take yours along. Such things are obsolete in today's hospitals and whatever they use instead requires a doctor's prescription. He could be off playing golf (mine ran in the Boston Marathon), and you'd have cold feet forever.

You can safeguard yourself against hepatitis by dropping by the hospital a couple of times well before O-Day, leaving a pint of your own good stuff on ice. If you go to the hospital for a pre-op work-up ahead of time, make sure your doctor clears your entry for the operation so the same tests won't be done again *routinely*—as you sign in.

Meet the doctor you have decided on and talk to him. If he won't talk to you and answer every single question you have written on your list, go somewhere else. Do this well ahead of time—not when the wheels are already turning and you are irrevocably scheduled.

Read up on the procedure being offered. Know what you are in for. Find out what your doctor's attitude is about painkillers. If he is paranoid about addiction, you will suffer because of his problem. Get a feel for his attitude toward patients. A doctor should be willing to answer your questions. When I was slated to have a cesarean section with my first baby I asked the

169

surgeon what would happen on the morrow. "Don't bother your little head. That's my worry." Do you think I worried? Sure I did, because I had no answers.

We have talked about how to survive a hospital, but there are also things to do *before* you get there.

How can you make an intelligent decision about surgery? You can ask a number of questions. First, ask about the surgeon. How experienced is he? You are entitled to know how many operations he has done, and if he is new at it, you must understand that you will be a learning experience for him. That's daring, but not sensible. You will be safer with someone who does them on a regular basis. If the doctor is evasive, go elsewhere.

Once you have settled on the surgeon you take the next step—check on the hospital. You need to know what the mortality rate is for your proposed surgery. Not too many people think about mortality at all, if it can be avoided. In this case it can't. According to Dr. George Crile, Jr. of the Cleveland Clinic, mortality rates for open heart surgery can vary from 5 to 30 percent, depending on the hospital. First, call the health director at the hospital where your surgeon operates and ask for that information. Next, call the county medical society, and they can tell you whether the rate is low or high. If it is high, go to another surgeon in a hospital with a better record.

Before you leap onto the operating table, look into alternatives. Is there another way to go? There are almost always alternatives, and while you are asking about them, find out what your chances are of a cure. What will you be like, and what will you be able to do after the opeation? Some operations are so deforming and debilitating that you might be better off as you are, at least for the time being. Dr. George Crile, Jr.'s book, *Surgery, Your Choices and Your Alternatives*, will be helpful to you (see the Sources section for details).

Last, but certainly not least, what is the fee going to be? If you think it is too high, call other hospitals and surgeons and ask for their rates. There is a reasonable average cost, and you need that information beforehand.

BED BALLET

Bed exercises are valuable when you are recuperating from an operation or laid up with something broken. They are fun anytime. If you are slated for physiotherapy, this would be acceptable.

Two people working in concert do better bed exercise than one person working alone. Music is essential, and a good waltz rhythm, lively and stimulating, gets the best results.

Pay 100 percent attention to the work at hand and don't talk. One person leads the exercise and the other follows. If possible, the person being exercised should close the eyes and relax.

Open Arms

To begin, grasp the arms at the wrists, and applying gentle pressure lift both arms up toward the ceiling. Keeping the pressure even, move the arms wide and return. After returning to the upward reach, carry the arms across the body. Do several, listening to the music for cues on when to change.

When the music's phrasing changes, change the movement—this time to overhead and back down to the sides. The next variation is to alternate the arms.

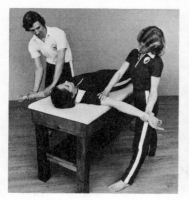 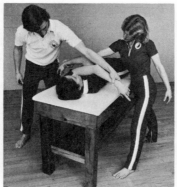 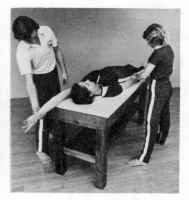

Bicycle

Babies love to have their knees bent, together and alternating. So do people who have to lie around all day unbent. Start with alternating, progress to double bends and return to alternating.

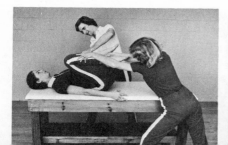 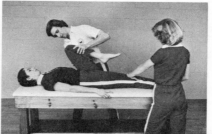

171

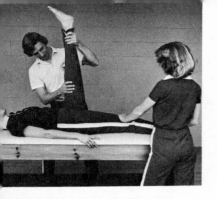

High Kicks

One exerciser holds one leg flat on the bed. The other exerciser raises the leg overhead, making sure to keep the knee straight. Alternate legs.

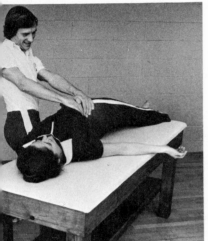

Side Pull

Reach across the body, grasping at the waist and pelvis. Pull those parts toward you and rock back to the resting position. The second operator is ready and on the beat pulls the other side of the body to the other side. Try never to leave the body of the person on the bed without contact with at least one hand. As long as the contact is kept no matter the action, the person being exercised feels secure.

At first the pull should be slow and easy. Take plenty of time and don't carry the pull to extremes. Let the body get used to a new condition. The person may have trigger points that need work. If there is pain find the points and erase them. Then you can go on to more vigorous work.

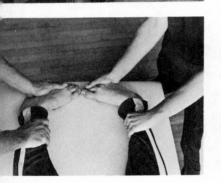

Feet In—Feet Out

One reason the heels of people long in bed get so sore is lack of circulation caused by trigger points in the legs, groin, and buttocks. Those should all be of concern and taken care of. Once the legs are clear, leg exercises will have more value.

Each operator holds one foot and ankle. Turn the toes inward until they touch. Next, without moving the position of the legs, turn the feet outward. Do several rotations before moving to the next step.

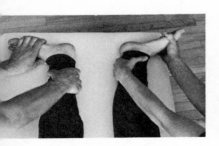

Leg Spreads

Start in the toe-in position with toes touching. As you rotate the feet outward this time, however, open the legs until the heels are about eighteen inches apart. Repeat the rotations of the feet while moving the legs inward and outward. Do several of these and week by week flexibility will improve and the stretch widen. Be sure to check the adductors for trigger points.

The Circle

Return to the arms. Each operator moves an arm to make a circle starting at the sides, carrying the arms outward and overhead, crossing in front of the face and ending at the sides. Without interrupting the flow, do three or four that way and then reverse the direction. This is excellent for shoulders and arms, upper back and chest.

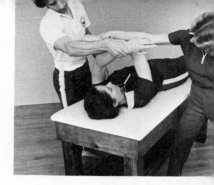

Sit-ups

The vigor with which this exercise is conducted is variable. A child with a foot in a cast, an athlete recovering from three months in traction, a housewife suffering exhaustion, and an elderly person whose legs are unstable all require different handling. Both operators support the head and back and bring the person to a sitting position, bending the upper body as far as is comfortable to stretch the back. He or she is then returned to the lying position and the action is repeated. After three or four sit-ups do a roll-back (next exercise).

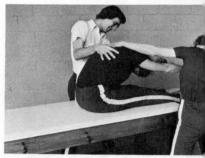

Roll-backs

Each operator grasps a bent leg just under the knee. Together they raise the knees and bring them toward the patient's forehead, lifting the seat slowly and carefully. Go no further than is comfortable. Backs that have been neglected in bed will complain like a rusty hinge at first. Check for trigger points and add a little distance at each session.

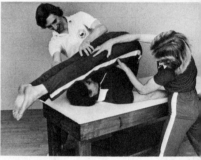

The Pull

Nothing but nothing feels better than the pull to a tired, bedridden body. One operator takes hold of the wrists and the other the ankles, pulling gently in rhythm to the music. As the music comes to an end each operator pulls against the pull of the other to stretch the person being worked over as hard as is wise considering the condition of the subject. Hold the steady pull about 15 to 20 seconds.

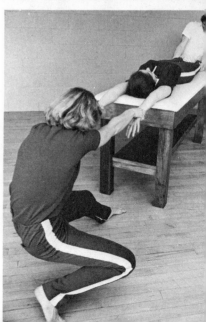

Solo Bed Exercises

Sometimes it is impossible to find two operators available at the same time. Rather than exercise first one side and then the other, the operator joins the subject on the table. Kneeling behind the person to be exercised, the operator is in complete control of the arms and torso. The sensation for the subject is similar to dancing while being led by an expert. The psychological gains are notable and in addition, if you are working with someone suffering from cerebral palsy or brain damage, someone who does not have complete control over the limbs, the safety factor is provided for.

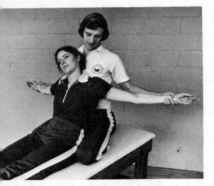

Open Arms

Taking both wrists in hand and using his body as a support, the operator opens both the subject's arms wide to the music and closes them. The close should be across the chest to stretch the upper back. The wide-open stretch stretches arms and chest. Do several and keep with the music. And even though the subject is in such condition as to *seem* not to respond, don't you believe that nothing is happening. If you can do this daily you will be amazed in a month at the changes in the subject. In most cases, you'll get good results in a week.

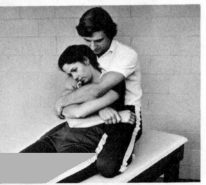

Close and Rock

Rock gently from side to side with the arms crossed over the chest. After several rocks try twisting a little to each side. It should be said here that music seems to provide control to muscles that defy their owners. Don't forget to check for trigger points.

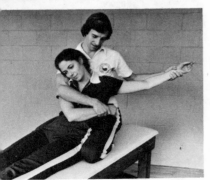

Alternating Arm Stretches

Pull first one arm out *and back* and then the other. This further stretches the arms and chest. It also provides a new dimension. You will find yourself making up new moves but don't worry if the moves are few. *You* are not "few"; you are many things to someone deprived of touch, warmth, companionship, and movement. Don't believe me, try it.

HOPELESS CASES? WE DON'T BELIEVE IT

This section is about recuperation from illness or injury. The chair exercises were invented 45 years ago when I smashed my pelvis on a ski slope before the days of physiotherapy. They have been used for just about any problem causing a person to be confined to a chair. At the least, they improve circulation, reduce fatigue, and are fun. At best, they are a bridge between sitting and walking. In one nursing home in New Hampshire, when the loudspeaker announces exercise in the lounge, there is a wheelchair traffic jam in the halls.

Alice is a student at the Bonnie Prudden School, and very soon she will be a certified exercise instructor as well as a myotherapist. We asked her to guide you through these next pages not only because she was injured and therefore knows something about the way back, but because she had given up trying to come back. Only months ago Alice was sent to us by one of the nation's largest insurance companies, labelled a "hopeless" case. Her hip had been broken and pinned. Infection set in and there were more operations, culminating in a total hip replacement. Years of suffering had passed, and the pain and disability persisted. Despair had set in for many reasons, and those reasons are what make Alice perfect for this chapter. First, her greenhouse work was over and that's what she knew how to do. She was nearing fifty. Who wants a fifty year old even if the job market wasn't glutted with kids just out of school with the latest skills? Her children were all grown and involved with their own lives. She would soon be living entirely alone. The house would be too big, but her life would be small, circumscribed by constant pain, inability to get around, and fear of tomorrow.

It took *one hour* of myotherapy to relieve much of the spasm that was preventing the surgeon's excellent job from working properly. It took two sessions to chase away despair and dispel her fear of coming unglued. The insurance company, no longer saddled with a "hopeless case," is helping with Alice's tuition. Now she no longer needs myotherapy; instead, she is equipped to provide it. Remember, the chair exercises are for people who are confined to chairs or who are uncertain of their footing, not just for "hippies." However, it will be interesting for those of you who have had total hip replacements to see how well they *can* work. Alice's replacement is on the left.

175

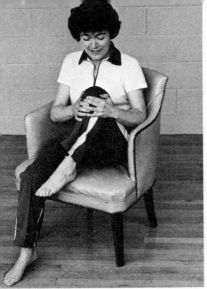

The Knee Lift, Assisted

Place both hands in front of the knee and lift as high as possible. This strengthens the arms and stretches the back. After doing this a few times with each leg, lift as before, but at the top of the lift remove your hands and try to maintain the lift for a few seconds and then lower slowly. Do four of these to a side, alternating legs. When this exercise is easy try the next one.

The Knee Lift, Free

Place your hands on the arms of your chair and bring the left knee as close to your nose as possible. This stretches the back and strengthens the abdominals. Alternate four to a side.

Knee Cross

Most people cross their knees without thinking about it. Some always cross the same one, without realizing it, because their torso is uneven. Some people can't cross their knees at all because they have trigger points in the gluteals, groin, and outer leg muscles. Don't lose the ability to do this simple movement. Keep the muscles clear of spasm. The spasms that prevent crossing can eventually prevent walking.

Slide your seat forward in the chair and lean back. Cross the left knee over the right and then alternate. Start with two or three and work up to sixteen. If there is pain in the back, groin, or thigh, check for trigger points. This exercise strengthens the legs and abdominals. When it becomes easy add the following.

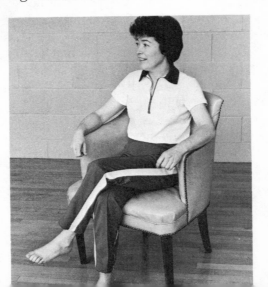

Knee Cross and Kick

Keep the same body position but each time you cross one knee over the other kick up as high as possible.

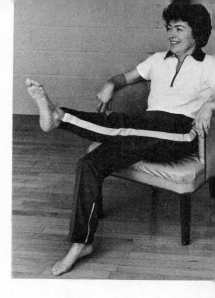

Knee Cross, Pull Up and Open

Cross the left knee over the right, bringing the foot over the thigh. Grasp your left foot and pull it up toward you to stretch the back, gluteals, and outer leg muscles. Next, swing the leg to the left and drape it over the arm of the chair. Then replace it on the floor. Alternate sides for four to a side. (That side drape is very restful.)

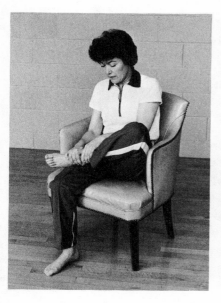
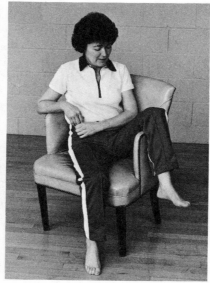

Neck Rest

Sit relaxed in the chair or stand at ease, and let your head fall forward. Let it hang for about five seconds while you try to let go wherever muscles in the neck, shoulders, or upper back resist. If there is even a slightly painful pull anywhere in the area, there are trigger points. Check with head, neck, and upper and lower back maps and have them erased. Roll your head slowly to the right side. If there is pain or tightness, check the sterno-

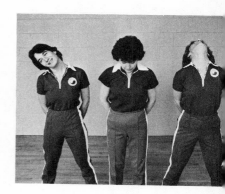

cleidomastoids (see Plate 6 in Appendix 1). Move your head and neck slowly back and forth just above your shoulder. Open your mouth and repeat the gentle rolling motion. Try to find tight areas and urge them to relax. Roll them to the left side and repeat the rolling motion. Finish by dropping the head forward and then tipping back. Open your mouth to ease neck muscles.

If you hear snaps, crackles, and pops, don't think arthritis. Think tight muscles, because that's what is causing the noise. When your neck, face, and head have been cleared of trigger points, silence will reign.

Feet In—Feet Out

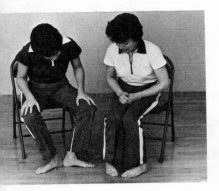

Place the feet parallel and rotate them inward, bringing the toes together. Next rotate them outward as far as possible. Start with about eight rotations to music and alternate with the next exercise, heel lifts, for several sets.

Heel Lifts

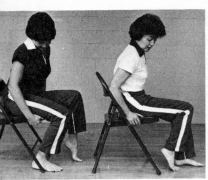

Place your feet flat on the floor and parallel. Keep the toes and ball of the left foot on the floor and raise the heel. Try to arch the foot and push the instep over the toes. Lower the foot and alternate feet for several bars of music. Long-second-toe holders, this is for you. If your feet are stiff, have them detriggered and massaged, and then use this exercise.

Toes Up–Toes Down

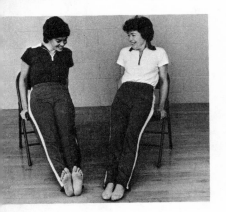

Slide forward until your seat is on the very edge of your chair. Lean back to rest your shoulders, and stretch your legs straight out in front. Keeping your feet together and parallel, press the soles of your feet flat to the floor. Then, with your heels still resting on the floor, pull your toes up toward your body as far as possible.

This exercise not only improves the flexibility of ankles and strengthens the legs, but aids the heart as it flushes the blood back up into the torso. So don't just sit there, move! Alternate several sets of toes up, toes down with the next exercise.

Toes Up–Toes Out

Stay seated with legs outstretched as you were. Rotate your toes inward as far as possible and then outward. Try to bring the outer edges of your feet to rest on the floor. This exercise stretches and strengthens the muscles of the ankles, legs, and feet. Do repetitions.

To increase the value of this exercise and the one just before, combine them to do foot circles. Press flat, rotate inward, pull up, rotate outward, and end with feet flat. Reverse the circles every four.

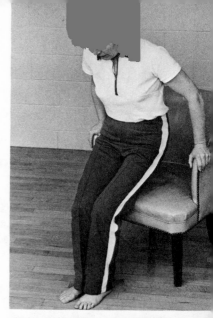

Seat Lift

Place your hands on the arms of your chair close to the front and straighten your arms to lift your seat into the air. Lower *slowly*, taking five seconds to accomplish the descent. Start with two and work up to six. This is a good arm strengthener. (If you have been incapacitated for some time and promised crutches by next Tuesday, start with this today. You'll need it.)

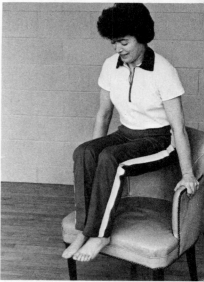

Seat Drop

Start at the top of the seat lift. Then bend the knees and raise the feet off the floor. Lower your body slowly to the sitting position on the chair. This comes after considerable work with the seat lift. The next step is to build the arm strength to lift yourself *up* from the sitting position to the top of the lift.

Back Stretch

Sit back in your chair and place your feet apart and flat on the floor. Keep your hands on the arms of your chair and lean forward to drop your head between your knees, or as close to that position as possible. Bounce your upper body downward three times and then sit up. Do three of those every time you think of it—and think of it often. It stretches the back and chest muscles.

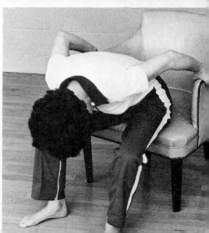

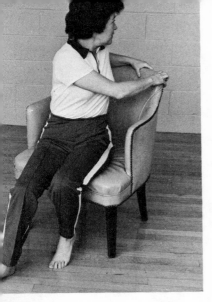

Waist Twist

Keep your feet well apart. Twist your upper body around to the left, bringing both hands as close to the back of the chair as possible. Swing to the right in the same manner. Alternate sides from four to eight times. This exercise loosens back muscles—just what a "hippie" needs. But then, so does everyone. It will also trim your waist and move things around inside as though they were being massaged.

Arm Arcs

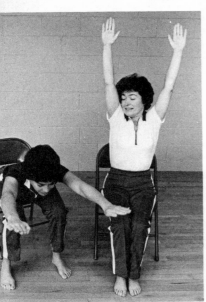

Slide forward in your chair placing your feet parallel and flat on the floor. Lean forward from your hips stretching your arms out in front. Sit erect and raise your hands straight overhead pressing your shoulders back. Next, open your arms wide and press back down in a wide arc. Do three. This exercise stretches the back, arms, chest, shoulders, axilla, and neck. If you had trigger points show up in any of these areas, this is an excellent exercise to use throughout the day to keep them at bay. Incidentally, this is the sit-up version of the circle in "bed ballet."

Upper-Torso Twist

Lean down between the feet and reach around behind the right leg to grasp the outsde of the right ankle with your right hand. Return to the erect position. Do the same movement to the other side. Next, reach down on the outside of the right knee with the left arm and reach around the back of the right leg to grasp the inside of the right ankle with the left hand. Repeat to the other side. Do four to a side. This exercise increases the flexibility of the upper torso, arms, and shoulders.

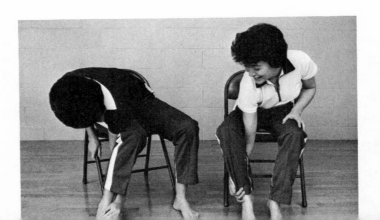

Body Lift

Move your seat forward in your chair and grasp the sides of the chair. Stretch your legs straight out in front pressing your feet flat to the floor and drop your upper body forward. Raise the entire body, arching the back and let your head fall backward. Hold the arched position for a slow count of three, and then slowly lower to the original sitting position. This exercise stretches the abdominal and chest muscles and strengthens the arms, upper back, and shoulders. Start with two and work up to six.

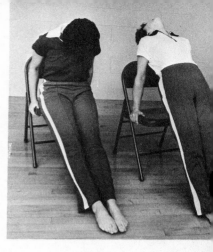

Snap and Stretch

This is the sitting version of the snap and stretch used in an exercise class and also after myotherapy for the chest muscles. Sit forward in your chair and raise bent elbows to shoulder level with hands crossed one over the other in front of your chest. Keeping the arms at shoulder level snap bent elbows back on the count of one. Return to starting position on two. Fling arms wide on three and return to start on four. Do eight.

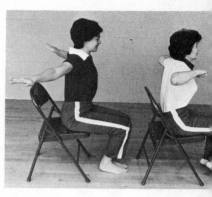

Push-ups

Be sure your chair is anchored against the wall so it cannot slip, and also be sure your feet are secure so that you cannot slip. Stand back from the chair (the distance will be greater as you improve). Grasp the front edge of the chair seat. Place your feet wide apart at first. This makes the exercise a little easier. Slowly lower your body into the let-down position. Then push up to the straight-arm position and return to the standing position. Place your hands in the small of your back, pressing head and elbows backward. Try to stretch your whole body. Start with two and work up to as many as you can manage.

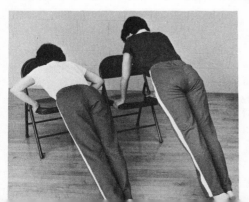

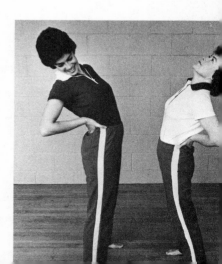

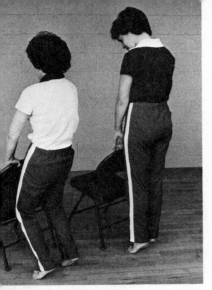

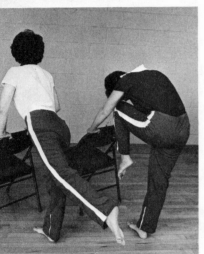

Pelvic Tilt Assisted

Stand with feet flat and hands resting on the chair back. Rise slowly on the toes tightening your abdominals and leg and seat muscles. Keeping your head down and seat tucked under, do a half knee bend. Straighten and return your heels to the floor. This exercise helps you to develop the pelvic tilt, so necessary to good posture and freedom from backache and fatigue. It also strengthens feet and legs and corrects sway back. Do three for a start and work up to ten.

Knee In–Leg Out

Start by standing behind the chair and grasping the back for support. Bring the left knee as close to your nose as possible. Swing the left leg backward and at the same time lift your head. Do four such in-out swings and four with the other leg. Do three sets. This exercise will stretch your back and abdominals and strengthen both areas as well. It is useful for improving your seat line and for resting a back that has been sitting at work too long.

Hugging Exercise

Hugging came about out of necessity. We had been doing a workshop at the Laconia State School in New Hampshire. Our participants were the handicapped residents. The higher functioning residents could follow us easily, but the severely handicapped could not. We tried the "hugging" in desperation, and it turned into a triumph. Be sure to have delightful slow music at first, and some good wild "rock" for the fast music. The "hugged" keep eyes closed.

Today the hugging series is used routinely, and not just with the handicapped. Our experiences at Laconia and elsewhere showed us that many people who had given up and were withdrawing into themselves came back. There was soon more comprehension, more reaction, more self-help. What was hugging all about? We soon found out.

We tried the series at our annual five-day workshop at Amherst College. It was a smashing success, but since no one was handicapped we added a fast piece in which the leg-lift exercise is featured and all the other movements speeded up. Hilarity! The first-graders in our public school classes would not

182

go home until hugged. We tried it at luncheon sites and workshops for the elderly. Tremendous! We tried it on teenagers. Wow! We tried it with little children visiting very old people in nursing homes. "Best thing that ever happened in here," said a nurse. We think there's nothing like "hugging."

Arms Out and Across

Stand behind the chair and take your partner's hands in yours. Ask him or her to close the eyes and just relax. When the music starts, open your arms taking your partner's along. Then carry the arms back and across. Do several and stay right with the music because the muscles of your partner are following the music. That's part of the magic; even in chairs they are all dancing. You can make circles too with the arms as in the "bed ballet."

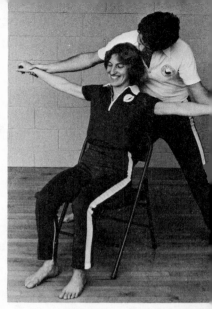

Push-down

Holding your partner's shoulders after having deposited his or her hands in the lap or over the sides, push the upper body forward and down and bring it back up. Keep your motions slow and steady and your hands firm and sure. We have come to believe that touch advertises what is coming and prepares the way. Do several.

Push-down with Twist

Still holding your partner's shoulders, twist the upper body to the left. Push down as before and return him or her to the erect position. Alternate sides several times. This is *very* helpful for people who must sit straight forward too much of the time.

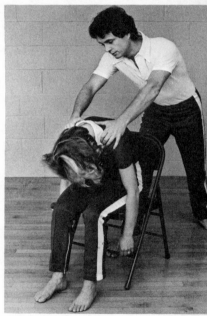

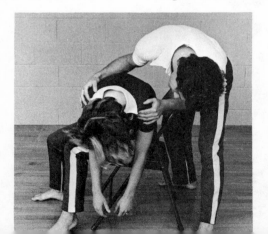

183

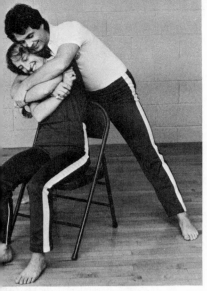

The Hugging

Pick up your partner's hands again, and placing your face next to his or her face, wrap your arms around the upper body holding your partner's arms inside your own. Rock left and right for several measures. Return to the arms exercise.

Chin-to-Head

Take your partner's wrists and lead both hands to your face. Rest your chin on the other's head and rock again as in the hugging. Go back to the push-down and then return to the hugging.

All these exercises can be done to slow music, which is advisable at first. After everyone knows what hugging is all about, then begin to pick up the beat.

Put on a fast, cheerful record, and begin by shaking your partner's shoulders back and forth to rhythm. Do this for a couple of bars and then change to twisting the shoulders, one forward and the other back. Then hold your partner's hands and move them as if you were conducting a band. Hug to a faster beat.

Pick up one leg with the knee bent. Put it down. Pick up the other leg, put it down. Alternate 4 times.

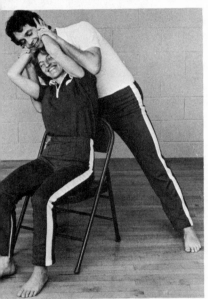

Leg Lift

Grasp the leg at the ankle and raise the straight leg. Lower and alternate 4 times with the other leg.

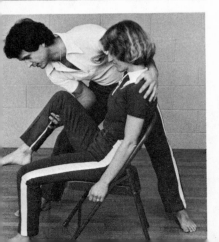

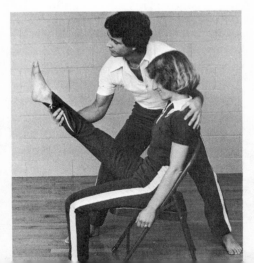

The Lift

Put your lower arms under the armpits of your partner and lift. Hold a second or two and then lower. Lift again and hold. There will be a great deal of laughter. This is a very funny feeling if your eyes are closed. Soon, everyone is talking up a storm. They can't believe the feelings. All good. What is hugging all about? It's holding, sharing, touching, and not only reaching out but drawing in. We need a lot of it, all of us.

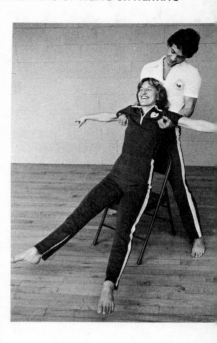

The Barre

The "barre" was born a year ago when my second hip was replaced. I watched the other patients stand by their doors, holding with trembling hands onto their walkers. Back in my room I was using my crutches to keep the weight off my new hip while I did dance steps to the music on my radio. Crutches were better for me because I was used to them, but they wouldn't be much better than walkers for those people in the hall. Maybe even less stable. There had to be an answer. The barre is the answer.

To make a barre you need two walkers, two pieces of pipe about eight feet long, a couple of sand bags, and some friction tape. Fasten the pipes to the walkers at two levels with the tape and hang the weight bags on the bottom rung for stability. Then crank up the record player. You have probably noticed that there are psychological aspects to almost everything we do, and the barre is no exception, nor are the uniforms we wear. A barre is for dancers, not for sickies. Standing in a hospital doorway in a wrap and slippers says you are sick. Working at a barre in warm-ups says something altogether different, and your subconscious hears it loud and clear. You are dancing. You must be better. Pretty soon you are.

When Alice and I do these exercises, it scares doctors half to death because they are sure the hip will come out of the socket. We have found that if the trigger points laid down by the diseased hip joints are erased, the muscles function very well. Then all that's left is to build strength and develop flexibility. These two qualities are essential for coordination, which is often thought to be lost after injury.

185

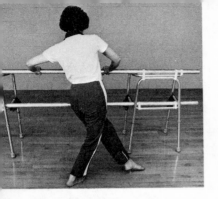

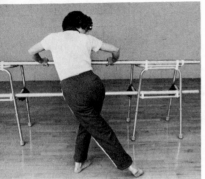

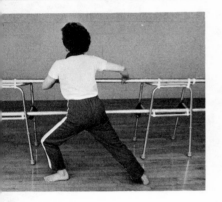

Toe Rises

Unused, feet weaken. They become unstable. Balance is impaired and the stage is set for a fall and a broken hip. First, take the trigger points from feet and legs and install the pads in the shoes of those with long second toes (see page 189). Then do the toe rises. Place the feet parallel and rise on the toes. Descend very slowly. Do four for a start and increase the number as strength increases. Use slow music or fast, but use music.

Cross-over

Stand on one foot, and to a good beat, cross the other over in front to touch the floor outside the standing foot. Return the crossing foot and then cross with the other. Alternate in this manner several bars. Then cross in back. Holding on to the barre gives stability, and also relaxes the whole body since you know you won't fall while getting into shape.

Charge

One of the facilities that is lost when hips, legs, or back are damaged, or when people who don't exercise regularly get old, is the ability to catch one's balance to the side. That must be regained, and also the ability to catch a backward fall.

Charge to the left and come back to the stand position and charge right. Alternate for eight, do another exercise, and come back for eight more.

Knee Bends

Several types of knee bends can be used: the half knee bend, assisted knee bend, and deep knee bend. All build muscle stretch and self-confidence.

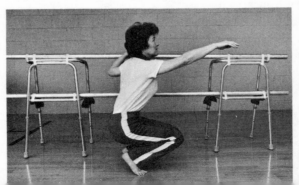

Hamstring Stretch

There are several ways to stretch hamstrings at the barre. Facing sideways and holding on with one hand and keeping the head up, bounce the upper body downward in eight easy bounces. This stretches the hamstrings in the legs.

Next, drop the upper body down in eight bounces to stretch the back. Alternate four times.

Facing the barre and holding on with both hands it is possible to stretch the back and hamstrings while also stretching the chest muscles.

In order to increase chest stretch, bounce with one hand on the upper barre and one on the lower.

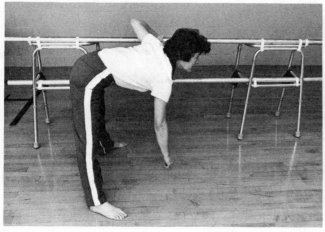
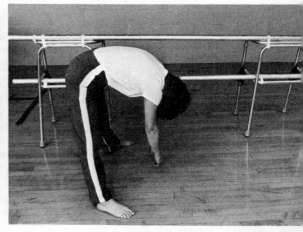
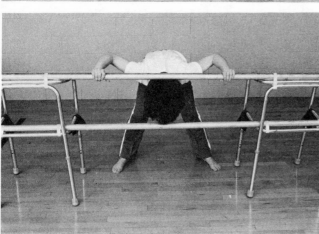
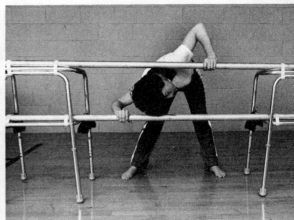

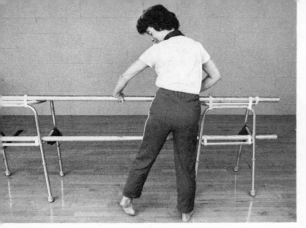 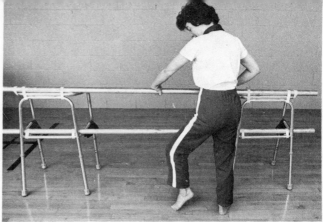

Hip Twists

If you want your body to move well you have to instruct it to move well, train it to move well, and then make it move. I hope by now you are convinced that, for your health's sake, you had *better* move.

Turn the foot inward and outward from the hip. Do eight with each leg for a start and work up as fast as you feel you can, without overdoing it.

Get Your Leg Up There

If you want to get rid of the habit of limping that pain gave you, you must improve your range. To achieve that, when you exercise you must do things way beyond what it takes to walk effortlessly and with grace.

Pick your foot up and set it on the bottom barre and then put it down. Alternate for four at first and work up to many.

Stretch that leg on the barre at first by standing and later by leaning forward toward the knee. (You won't do this until your body says it's all right.)

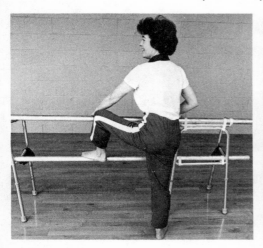 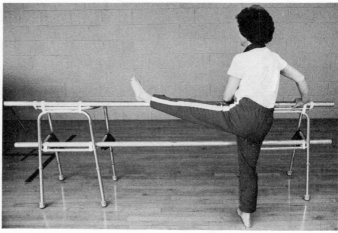

Holding onto the barre with both hands

> *Bounce to a beat*
> *Stretch to a beat*
> *Dance to a beat. Walk to a beat . . .*
> *Jump to a beat.*

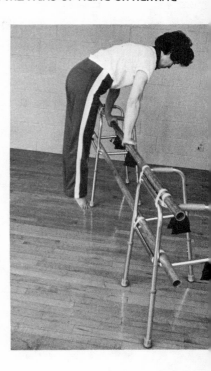

And don't be afraid. Your body will tell you what you can do.

The best surgeon in the world, doing the best job in the world on your hip, your knee, and all those places that hurt, will only succeed if you help by building the muscles that move the joints the surgeon provided. What happens now is up to you.

Aqua-Ex

My Japanese bath (see illustration page 95) is deep enough and wide enough and long enough and warm enough for the swimming lessons I once planned for my grandchildren. That was before my children were even out of school. I never suspected that it would become a life-saving well, filled with pain-relieving and hope-offering waters.

After myotherapy, after operations, warm water relaxes muscles and allows one to defy gravity and establish or re-establish rhythms forgotten or blotted out by pain.

For shoulders and arms we use arm exercises. Swimming motions, circles under water, pushing down, and pulling up. Almost any movement will do. For legs and hips, water is especially appropriate.

Aqua-Ex can be done at a public pool if it isn't too cold, and many Y's do have courses called "Aqua-Ex." The instructors, however, do sometimes forget that they are using water as a form of resistance and that some exercises belong only in the gym. The following program, photographed on dry land, is the one we use with considerable success at the myotherapy institute.

The Toe Bounce

Walk through the water to some music with a good, brisk tempo. Bounce down on your heel and right up onto the toe. This action will do a number of things, from maintaining strength in the feet and lower legs to keeping down the swelling that all too often accompanies inactivity. Bounce along about 20 steps.

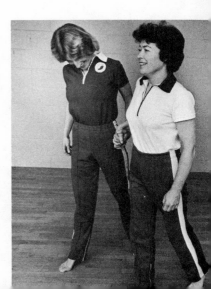

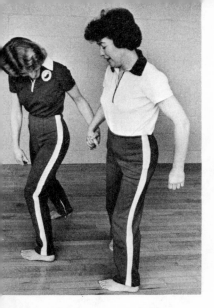

Toes In—Toes Out

You have already met this exercise in its varying forms. In the pool you can walk eight steps turned in and then eight turned out. Alternate like that all the way across, if you like. Or perhaps four in and four out. It doesn't matter so long as it pleases you, because then you will do it.

The Twist

Turning the whole lower body with each step helps maintain the torso muscle tone and keeps the waist slim during the time of enforced inactivity.

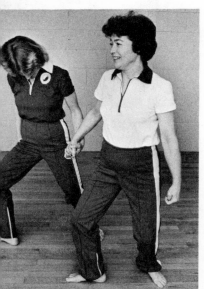

High Knee Lifts

High knee lifts walking through water strengthen the quadriceps, the great muscles of the thighs.

Goose Step

This too works the quads, which stabilize the knees, provided they harbor no trigger points.

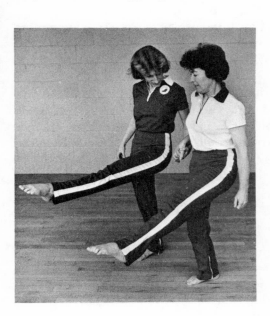

Apart-Together Jumps

Like jumping jacks but without the arm action. Keeps the adductors and vastus lateralis in good working order.

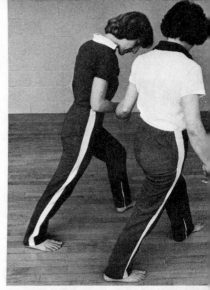

Hip Rotations

Do the same hip twists you did at the barre, but hopping onto the other foot as you twist.

Walking Backward

This exercise works the gluteals and the muscles in the backs of the thighs.

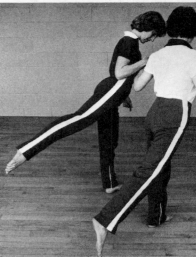

Kick Back

This exercise does the same thing as walking backward, only more so.

The simple act of walking in water up to your shoulders is a strength builder where walking along the beach might be too much. Walk forward, backward, and sideways. Water is resistance, and muscles need resistance. The mind, however, must be pleased or the exercises will not be done. So find your particular water hole, turn on the music, and dance.

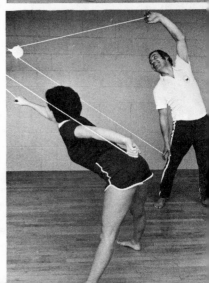

The Pulley

One more gadget to help you get back into the world is the pulley. The pulley is to be found at your local friendly hardware store, and there is nothing fancy about it. A plastic pulley (get a nice big one), twelve feet of quarter-inch nylon rope (get the best grade, after all, it's for *you*), two dowel handles (we cut ours from old broom handles). Fasten the pulley to something immovable. One solution is a six-inch length of thin nylon cord with a knot in it and laid over the top of a door. When the door is closed, the knot is on the outside while you and your pulley are inside.

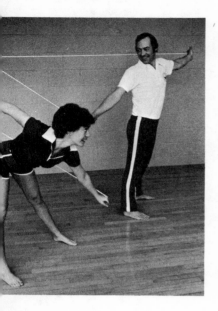

Use the pulley without resistance at first and then start giving one arm resistance with the other. If you have to start from scratch after injury, the pulley can be fastened to a hospital overhead frame, or the foot of a bed. You can use it from a chair. The principal thing is—use it. It will help shoulders and arms, upper back and chest. Pull your pulley to music.

Incidentally, for post-mastectomy the pulley is a must. I invented it for a friend in 1962. Take the trigger points from your scar tissue and begin.

To Ward Off Pain— Test Your Fitness, Improve Your Fitness

10.

The Kraus-Weber Minimum Muscular Fitness Test for Key Posture Muscles is medically valid. It takes only 90 seconds to give and requires no computation. You either pass or flunk, and it provides lots of valuable information.

The K-W Test was developed at the Columbia Presbyterian Posture Clinic in New York City. It was designed to test the function of muscles on a minimum level. We used it to prove that the physical fitness of American children in the forties and fifties was probably the lowest in the entire world.

Tests 1 and 2 are for minimum abdominal strength. Without at least a minimum level of strength, proficiency in sport or childbearing is virtually impossible. If the abdominals are weak, their work will have to be taken over by the iliopsoas, the muscle that attaches to the spine at about waist level and to the lesser trochanter in the thigh. And it never pays to overwork a muscle that ties into and may pull on the spine.

The test for the psoas is number 3. Tests 4 and 5 are devoted to the minimum strength of the upper and lower back muscles. The last, Test 6, is the only test that checks on flexibility. Number 6 tests the flexibility of the back muscles and hamstrings.

Coordination depends on a combination of strength plus flexibility. Since everything we do, from walking to skydiving, depends on coordination, obviously we need both strength and flexibility.

The minimums set up apply to that level of strength and flexibility needed for daily living. Nothing special like sport, a war, or having a baby. Just plain, simple, daily living.

You will soon see that freedom from back pain also depends on this vital combination.

A study was done at Columbia Presbyterian Hospital in New York City by Doctor Sawnie Gaston. He and his group gave a battery of tests to thousands of people suffering with back pain. Blood tests, urinalysis, orthopedic tests, neurological tests, psychiatric tests . . . and the K-W Test. Over 80 percent of the subjects had no anatomical pathology at all. The only test they failed was the one for minimum muscle strength and flexibility. When they brought their muscles into better condition, the pain went away. It was as simple as that.

From that study we learned that there is a fitness level below which the average human cannot fall without courting pain.

The children entering school in the forties and early fifties had a 54 percent failure rate on the K-W Test. We have confirmed the tests over the years. Children coming into the school system now are up to an 85 percent failure rate in many schools, and in some areas it runs as high as 100 percent. The potential for future pain in these depressing figures is mind boggling.

Since you are reading this book, there is more than a little hope for you and yours in the battle against pain. The first thing you need to know is just where each of you stands on the K-W fitness scale. You should also begin to look at your family's posture and encourage them to observe yours. Are your shoulders hunched or rounded? Have you got a swayback? Do your feet turn in, or out? Like a K-W Test failure, those posture faults aren't normal.

You will need a card such as the one that follows here for each person, and you should test regularly at given times each year. For children it should be done when they enter school in September. If you send "healthy" children to school who are able to pass the test, and you get back unhealthy kids who cannot pass the test by Christmas, scream bloody murder at the PTO meeting, at the school board, and at whoever is responsible for "phy.ed." Then put the children in the best dancing school, gymnastic school, swim school, riding school, soccer school, or ski school available, after classes.

The Kraus-Weber (K-W) Tests

Six tests for minimum muscular fitness.

Function and posture. Check often.

Name_____Age _____

BOX A			
Date			
A+			
A−			
P			
UB			
LB			
FL			

BOX B			
Substitution			
Leading elbow			
Arch			
Scoliosis			
Round shoulders			
Swayback			
Pigeon toes			
Turn out			

THE TESTS

Here are the instructions on how to administer and score the tests. You should also take time to look for postural conditions such as round shoulders, swayback, pigeon toes, and feet that turn out. Make note of these conditions in the boxes on the K-W card, and use myotherapy and exercise to correct them. (See the index for appropriate sections in this book.)

Test 1: Abdominals Plus Psoas (A+)
PURPOSE: To test the strength of the abdominal muscles plus the psoas (hip flexors), which are inside the pelvis.
POSITION: Lying supine with hands clasped behind the head and legs straight. Hold the feet down with strong pressure.
COMMAND: "Keep your hands behind your neck and roll up into a sitting position." If the subject sits up no matter with what contortions, the test is passed. Put a check next to A+ in Box A. If the test is passed with difficulty, add a small *c* to the check. If the subject cannot sit up, enter 0.

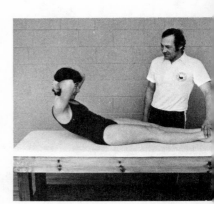

195

If the subject cannot roll up with a rounded back, but jerks up with a straight back, put a check next to "Substitution" in Box B. That means the muscles are not working all along their length, and substitution, which is abnormal, is going on.

If the subject comes up with the torso twisted, so that one elbow leads the other, put an *R* or *L* (for right or left) next to "Leading elbow" in Box B. It means that the muscles on one side of the torso are stronger than those on the other, and the weaker side must be strengthened. Uneven strength causes an uneven pull and may lead to scoliosis (spinal curvature).

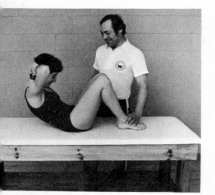

Test 2: Abdominals Minus Psoas (A−)
PURPOSE: This is a further test for the abdominals and a truer abdominal test than A+. Slide the heels up toward the seat. The bent-knee position lessens the assisting power of the psoas, throwing most of the strain on the abdominals rather than the spine.
POSITION: Same as for Test 1, but with knees bent.
COMMAND: "Keep your hands behind your neck and roll up into a sitting position." If the sit-up is successful put a check next to A− in Box A. If impossible, 0. Don't forget to add a *c* if difficult. Watch for same clues as for Test 1.

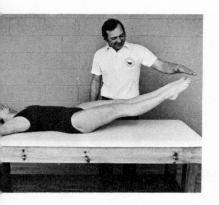

Test 3: Psoas (P)
PURPOSE: To test the strength of the psoas, or hip flexors. (These muscles are developed by running, skipping, and jumping.)
POSITION: Same as for Test 1.
COMMAND: "Keep knees straight and raise both legs up until your feet are about eight inches off the table (or floor)." Indicate that spot, as many people can't judge distances. "Hold while I count." Count ten seconds which is easily done by adding a three syllable word to each number. Kids like "chim-pan-zees."

If the hold is for the full ten seconds, enter a check in Box A, next to P. If the full ten was not held, enter the number of the second when the feet touched the table.

Ideally there should be no hitch in the pelvic area when the legs are lifted and no extreme arch in the back. If these signs are in evidence enter a check next to "Arch." It means that the psoas is weak and a swayback may be developing, in which case corrective exercise, discussed later in this chapter, is in order.

Test 4: Upper Back (UB)
PURPOSE: To test the strength of the upper back muscles.
POSITION: Prone, over a pillow or rolled towel. This gives the body the appearance and function of a seesaw. Hands are clasped behind the head and feet held down.
COMMAND: "Keep your hands behind your head. Raise your head, chest and shoulders as though you were a plane taking off. Hold that while I count." Don't let the subject arch unduly as this makes the test too easy; just have the chest clear the table. The count is ten seconds and the results are handled as in Test 3.

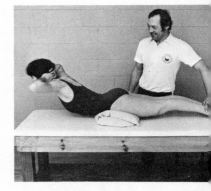

Test 5: Lower Back (LB)
PURPOSE: To test the strength of the lower back.
POSITION: Prone over pillow, head resting on arms, upper back held down.
COMMAND: "Lift up your legs, but don't bend your knees. Hold your legs up while I count." Again the count is for ten seconds and the results are handled as in the previous two tests.

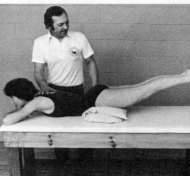

Test 6: Flexibility (FL)
PURPOSE: To test the flexibility of the back and hamstring muscles. This is the only test for flexibility. It is highly important, as inflexibility seems to relate to stress, and where there is stress there is poor climate, and where there is poor climate, there is danger of injury and pain.
POSITION: Stand with feet together, knees held straight, and arms at sides. There is to be no warm-up or bouncing stretches.
COMMAND: "Keep your knees straight and lean down very slowly. Lean down and try to touch the floor with your fingertips. If you can, stay there while I count to three."

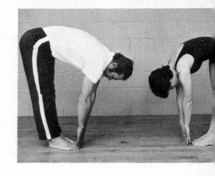

If the subject could not get down to touch, under FL enter a minus whatever number of inches were between fingers and floor. If the fingers just touched, enter *T* for touch. Touch is passing.

There are flexibility exercises later in this chapter, under Tried and True Exercises and Stretch Exercises. If the subject flunked Test 6, he or she will need all of them. For your work with myotherapy, however, you will want to know the location of the trigger points that are shortening the muscles. Have the

197

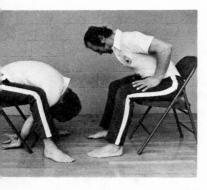

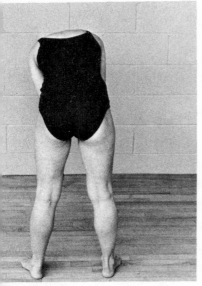

subject sit on a bench or the edge of a chair and with knees apart, try to press the head down between the knees. If the test was failed but the head goes way down like David's on the left here, then the tightness will be in the backs of the legs and the hips. If, however, the head can't come anywhere near the knees, the trigger points will be in the back. If the head and knees touch but just barely, then it will be 50-50, and a total search is in order.

There is one more important use for Test 6, and that is in the search for scoliosis. Many young people have curvatures for years before they are discovered. To find it early, one must look. Have the subject stand with feet apart for balance, knees straight. Lower the upper body slowly downward. You stand behind in a half crouch and watch the level of the back. If at any time one side rises higher than the other, you have scoliosis on your hands. Enter a check next to "Scoliosis" in Box B on the K-W test cards. A trigger point search as for back pain is indicated and then a complete exercise program.

Failure to pass Test 6 is usually an indication that the subject is not getting enough physical outlet to balance the stress he or she lives with, or that whatever physical outlet is being pursued is doing damage to both back and leg muscles. The flexibility exercises provided in this chapter should be done not just daily but several times every day.

Poor coaching is often responsible for the tight hamstrings noted in athletes. Few coaches seem to understand the relationship of flexibility to safety during the unpredictable stresses that are part of all spike sports like football, basketball, baseball, and so on. A falling body landing across the backs of a forward's legs in a pileup, or the shock resulting when ski tips hit a submerged log, can cause muscles to spasm. If muscles are tight to begin with and can't give, the spasm could be so acute as to sever completely the Achilles tendon.

Among other disadvantages, tight hamstrings can even contribute to poor running time. Let's suppose that Johnny has made the track team. He has a good build for running and plenty of motivation, but his flexibility test registers a −6 inches. If touching the floor is considered minimum, Johnny is six inches shy of that minimum with each leg. This means that for each two strides he gets a foot less distance than the boy who can touch. Another boy on the team, Earl, can not only turn in the minimum score, he can stand on a box and reach down over the side for three additional inches. With every two strides he gets six inches more than the boy who was just passing. Matched stride for stride, Johnny and Earl, equal in height, build, and motivation, are not equal in performance. Earl has a foot and a half advantage every two strides.

There is an additional danger for serious athletes, the ones who go to college on athletic scholarships, for example. They *have* to win if they want to stay in school. They have to practice and they have to stress their bodies mightily all four years. That sets up not only the trigger points but the tense climate of competition. The triggering mechanism could be provided by the explosive start off the blocks. Johnny might pull up lame a few yards later.

Childbirth is hardly a sport, but it does come under the heading of extreme physical effort. If inflexibility is present, it makes the whole job more difficult. Should weak abdominals also be part of the picture, labor will be accompanied by back pain and pain will accompany the mother when she leaves the hospital.

If you failed any of the K-W tests, this is the time to start your special exercise program. Do these corrective exercises as often as you can fit them into your day. Until you are proficient with these you will find all the other exercises in this chapter difficult. Continue these exercises until you can pass all six tests.

Before doing these exercises, it's a good idea to spend a minute doing the warm-up waist twists shown in the exercise section.

CORRECTIVES FOR THE K-W ABDOMINAL TESTS

Roll-downs and Sit-ups

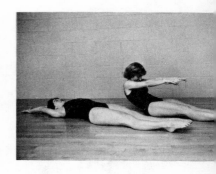

1. Sit on the floor with feet and arms stretched out in front of you. Drop your head, round your back and roll very slowly down until you are at rest. If you can, come up the same way. If you cannot, then stretch your arms on the floor above your head and pretend you are holding a basketball. Sit up as hard and fast as possible, throwing the imagined basketball across the room. If even that is not possible, simply do the first roll-down several times daily until you build the strength to roll up.

199

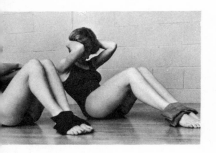

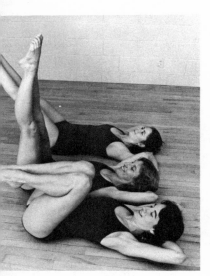

2. When you can get up with your arms stretched out in front of you, start your roll-downs with arms across your chest and then come up with arms stretched out in front of you. Work for the time you can also roll up with folded arms. When you can manage that, advance to the next, more difficult exercise, bent-knee sit-ups.

3. Bend your knees for the roll-down and put either a weight on your feet or your feet under a chair. By bending your knees, you cut out the help from the powerful psoas muscles and are forced to use your abdominals even more than before. By doing this you also safeguard your back. The psoas muscles attach at your spine and the leg bone called the lesser trochanter. If you do straight-leg sit-ups without the help of your arms, you force the psoas to overwork and pull on the spine. This can (and does) cause backache.

Cross your arms over your chest and roll very slowly down and come up the same way if you can. If not, come up with arms outstretched. Repeat this exercise until you can come up with arms folded and then advance to the hardest exercise in the series.

4. Place your hands behind your head while sitting in the bent-knee position. Roll slowly down and as slowly up again. If you can't come up with your hands behind your neck, come up with them across your chest. Do the roll-downs until you have the strength to come up with your hands behind your head. At this point you pass the minimum abdominal test. That doesn't mean stop there. That means doing ten such roll-downs twice daily from now on as part of your regular routine.

CORRECTIVE FOR THE K-W PSOAS TEST

Spine-down stretch

If you were unable to pass Test 3, or had difficulty in holding your legs up for the full ten seconds, or found that your back was unduly arched, the following exercise will correct the condition.

Lie on your back with knees bent and resting above your abdomen. You will find that your spine is pressed flat to the floor. Keep it there at all times.

Raise your legs straight into the air. At this point you will have no trouble keeping your spine down. Drop your legs back to the rest position.

The second time you extend your legs lower them about 6 inches nearer the floor. Retract to the rest position. Keep extending and retracting, lowering your legs a few inches each time until you can no longer keep the spine down. At that point, go back to the angle of extension when you still had full control over the spine. Do ten. This exercise should be done twice daily. Ultimately you will be able to extend your legs an inch or two above the floor while maintaining a perfectly flat back. This is an excellent exercise for those who have a swayback, medically known as lordosis.

CORRECTIVE FOR THE K-W UPPER AND LOWER BACK TESTS

Prone Arm and Leg Lifts

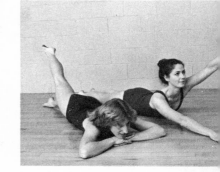

1. If you failed Test 4, lie prone on the floor with arms and legs outstretched. Raise first the left arm and then the right, being careful not to roll the upper body from side to side. Alternate for eight with each arm and do three sets daily.

2. If you failed Test 5, lie prone on the floor and raise the right leg as high as possible while keeping the knee straight. Alternate with the left for eight lifts with each leg. If this exercise is difficult or causes discomfort, place a pillow under the hips to prevent hyperextension. Check for trigger points in the gluteals, lower back, and groin. Do three sets daily.

CORRECTIVE FOR THE K-W BACK AND HAMSTRING FLEXIBILITY TEST

Back and Hamstring Stretch

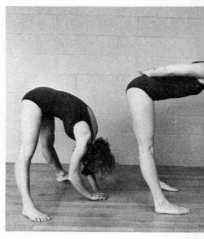

To gain sufficient flexibility to pass Test 6, place the feet wide apart and be sure to keep the legs straight. Clasp your hands behind your back, and keeping your head up, lean forward from the hips. Bounce your upper body downward in eight short, easy bounces. Repetition, not strain, will accomplish results, so don't push hard. Let gravity do the work. Do eight in the center, eight to the right, and eight to the left. Then allow the upper body to relax and hang down toward the floor. Do not force. Repeat the same easy bounces, eight center, eight right, and eight left.

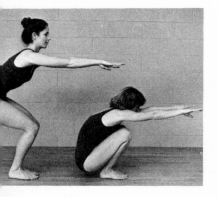

To improve the flexibility of the lower leg do half knee bends with heels tight to the floor. (You can even do some of these in the shower.) When you are able, do deep knee bends the same way (not in the shower).

Remember, tightness in the hamstrings is aggravated by stress. The more tension your day holds, the more you will need these exercises.

YOUR BASIC FITNESS PROGRAM TO KEEP PAIN AWAY

Myotherapy has made it not only possible to erase pain, but in most instances, easy. But that isn't the end of the problem. Now it's up to you to keep pain at bay. Unless you now get yourself into shape and stay that way, the pain will return. So let's start moving those muscles.

Warm-up Exercises

Muscles that have been in spasm for a time have developed bad habits. They become used to their shortened condition and tend to return to that condition from time to time. The best insurance against this is stretch exercise. Stretch, however, should never be attempted before a a proper warm-up. So, always start with easy warm-up exercises. In this program, easy exercises are preceded by the letter A.

The warm-up exercises should also be done by anyone who has been injured in sports or accidents, or by age or occupation, and by anyone intending to engage in sports, whether they be as undemanding as golf or as strenuous as dance, football, or high diving. And they should be done first. Stretch exercises are not warm-ups, and starting with stretch may well throw your muscles back into spasm.

Any exercise in this fitness program that is intermediate in difficulty will be preceded by the letter B. Do not attempt it until you feel comfortable with the A exercises. Difficult exercises will be preceded by the letter C. Advanced exercises, which should be done only by those in shape who are preparing for a sport, will be preceded by a D.

Even if your own workout at first is the correctives for the K-W Test, do a few of the warm-ups first. The only exceptions should be the side-lying exercise provided in the backache section, the cat back-old horse, and any other exercise called for in connection with specific pain erasure in this book. These can be done without doing the warm-ups first since they serve as warm-ups themselves. The exercises provided in this book have been tested for many years on both healthy and damaged people. They work. Many other forms of exercise do not. If you want to try other exercises after you are fine again and healthy, and in shape, go ahead. But don't experiment until you know you are fine.

Use music, brisk and of your choice.

A. *The Swim*

Stand with feet well apart for balance. Keeping the legs straight, bend forward from the hips. Use an overarm swim stroke. Alternating your arms, do eight strokes to the right, eight left and eight center. Repeat this set three times. Reach out as far as possible on each stroke and keep the knees straight. This works for shoulder and arm strength and shoulder and hamstring flexibility.

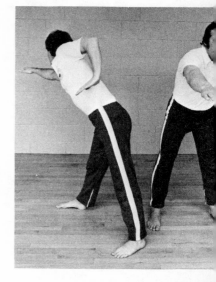

A. *Thigh Shift*

The safest way to exercise is with variety. Never spend longer than 20 seconds at a time on one area. Alternate with other parts of the body. You just used your arms, now shift to legs. Stand with feet apart and somewhat turned out. Keeping both heels flat on the floor, bend the left knee. Look down and be sure the knee covers your toes. If you can see your toes outside your knee your foot is inverting. Move your knee outward. Return to erect position and then bend the left knee, shifting the weight to the left thigh. Alternate legs for eight shifts. This exercise strengthens the leg muscles and therefore the knees. It stretches the backs of the lower legs. Go lower as strength improves.

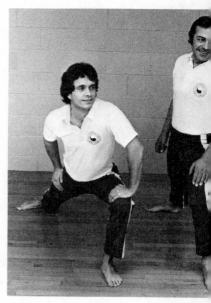

A. *Waist Twist*

Stand with feet well apart and hold bent arms at shoulder level. Twist the upper body all the way around to the right and then to

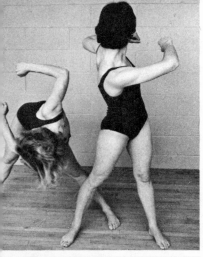

the left. Set up a good rhythm and start with 16 twists and work up to 30. By following the backward flung hand with your eyes, you will also improve the range of your neck. This exercise works all the muscles in your torso, groin, abdominals, and chest. It has the bonus of reducing both waist and abdominal area.

A. Right-Angle Twist

Feet well apart and the upper body held at right angles to the floor. Keep your head still so that your upper body may twist against the two set ends of the spinal column. Continue the same arm motion as in the waist twist. Start with 20 and work up to 50. This exercise also works the entire torso, strengthening the upper back and chest muscles while mildly stretching arm, back, and hamstring muscles. It also slims the waist.

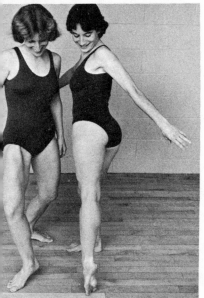

A. Hip Twist

With arms relaxed turn the left foot inward as far as possible. Bring the hip around as well. Then twist the foot, leg and hip outward. Repeat the rotation with each leg slowly, pressing open and closed as hard as you can. After eight slow rotations, double your time and do 16 to each side. This is an excellent hip exercise. It also strengthens the muscles in the upper leg and the gluteals. It is a must for low back problems.

A. Back Stroke

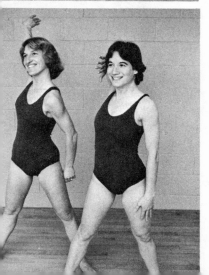

Place the back of the right hand on your right cheek, pressing the elbow back as far as it will go. Hold the elbow in the stretched position and swing the hand up, back, and down to complete a circle. Keep the shoulders facing front. Alternate eight with each arm. This exercise improves the range of the shoulders, stretches the pectorals, works against round back, improves upper back strength. Since many people do not really know what their bodies are doing, a good investment would be a full-length mirror so that you can see rather than feel whether your shoulders are really back.

A. Torso Shift

Stand with feet apart and arms extended to the sides. Pretend you are standing in a closet two feet wider than your arm reach. Keep the hips absolutely still and the shoulders level. Reach with the right hand to touch the imaginary wall at your right, then shift the upper body to touch the left wall. Start with 8 shifts done slowly and work up to 30 at the lively tempo. This exercise separates the upper from the lower torso and is excellent for those with scoliosis (curvature of the spine). It will help improve performance in all sports.

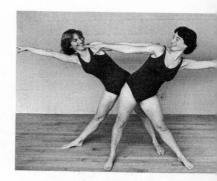

A. Pelvic Tilt Standing

Pretend you are a small child standing with feet apart, knees bent, hands on knees, and seat pushed out in back. If someone were to walk up behind you and swat your seat with a paddle, and it was against the rules to jump, let go of your knees, or straighten your legs, what would you do? You would tuck your pelvis under and tighten your unprotected posterior into a hard knot. Hold that position for a slow count of five and then push your seat out back to the point where you started. Do eight. This exercise is essential for posture, athletics, sex, and freedom from back pain. It strengthens the abdominals and lower back muscles. If the problem is impotence or frigidity, as mentioned in connection with old coccyx injuries, as soon as the trigger points have been removed, start this exercise. Use it often every day.

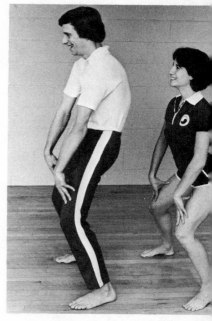

A. Lateral Stretch

Stand with feet apart and place the left hand on the left thigh and the right straight up overhead. Lean the upper body and raised arm to the left as you slide the left arm down the leg to the knee level. Holding this position, bounce the upper body downward in four short, easy bounces. Then do the same to the other side.

At this point we should say something about static stretch as opposed to bounces. The static-stretch fad has been around several years. It may last another few. Flexibility bouncing has been around for several thousand through dance. We have found it safer, more effective, more fun, and more valuable when it comes to getting muscles in shape.

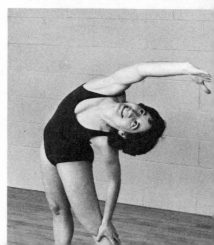

The lateral stretch improves the range of the torso and shoulders. It helps release spasms in the latissimus dorsi as well as every muscle down to the feet on both sides of the body. It strengthens the abdominals.

A. Snap and Swing

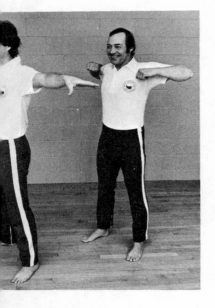

Start with the feet apart and elbows bent and held at shoulder level. Snap the elbows back for a count of one. Then return to the starting position for the count of two. Swing the arms open and back for the count of three and return to the starting position for the count of four. Be sure to keep the arms at shoulder level at all times. Do eight sets. This exercise is another good one for round shoulders. It opens the chest to improve the capacity of the lungs. Doing aerobic work to improve the lungs will be a waste if the lungs have nowhere to expand because they are strapped down with tight muscles. This exercise also strengthens the upper back, stretches arm muscles, and improves shoulder range.

B. Walk-outs

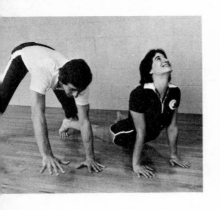

Start in the standing position with feet apart. Without bending the knees, lean forward from the hips and place one hand on the floor. Walk your hands forward for three counts but do not move the feet. On the fourth count, when the body is stretched full out, press the pelvis downward with a sharp movement, but do not bend your arms. Walk your hands back for two counts and allow the last two counts for standing straight. Do two at the start and work up to eight. This exercise strengthens arms, hands, shoulders, back, and abdominals. It will stretch the groin, the abdominals, and the hamstrings.

C. Knee Bends

Older people who did many knee bends in their youth know them to be an excellent exercise. Younger people are not so fortunate. In the sixties a controversy arose over knee bends that caused a great deal of confusion and contributed to a great number of knee injuries. A study was done on the knee injuries suffered by a small group of football players and an even smaller group of weight lifters. All of these players had suffered knee injuries when in the deep knee-bent position, duck walks for the football players and squats for the weight lifters. The report that came out of the study held that deep knee bends caused ligament injuries and must not be done by anyone, even children. I believe this to be an erroneous conclusion. Football and weight lifting lay down trigger points in leg muscles, setting them up for spasm when a triggering mechanism is encountered. For the men in the study the triggering mechanism was the knee bend following years of repeated strain and injury.

All joints including knees, should be provided with full range of motion. Once your legs have been detriggered, bend them.

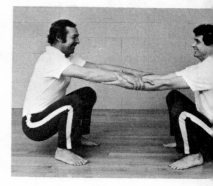

Stand with legs either together or slightly apart, heels flat on the floor. Stretch your arms forward at shoulder level and drop slowly down into a deep knee bend. If you have trouble keeping your heels on the floor, grasp a partner's forearms for support or hold onto the two handles of an open door. Those who can, start with 5 and work up to 50 daily.

This exercise strengthens the massive thigh muscles controlling the knees, and the tibialis anterior which affects foot action. It also stretches the heel cords.

Tried and True Exercises

You are now, we hope, free of pain and warmed up. So let's get on with our conditioning exercise to fight off future pain. Remember to look for the letter that assures you that the exercise isn't too hard, so far. A for easy, B for intermediate, C for difficult, and D for advanced.

A. Pelvic Tilt, Sitting

Sit on the floor and clasp your hands in front of your knees. If you have one of those tailbones that aches after the first half hour at the board meeting or movie show, get a bath towel. Fold it in half. Take the two edges and fold them into the middle. Fold the outside edges once more to the middle, and you will have a cushion with a space running down the center. Sit on it so that the tailbone rests in that space.

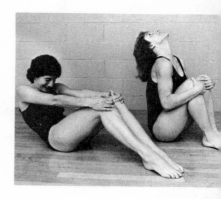

Lean back as far as you can without tipping over. Drop your head and round your back. Tighten the abdominals, gluteals, and levator ani. (See Plate 19 in Appendix 1.) To tighten those muscles contract as you would to prevent urination and defecation. Hold for a count of four, and then sit up as straight as you can and tip your head back. Get your back absolutely straight, even arch it if possible. Do eight.

A. Side Drop

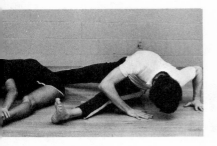

Start with the legs spread wide. Drop your upper body first to the left side, resting your weight on your left hand which is placed on the floor under the shoulder. That stretches the chest, shoulder, and underarm. Swing back to the sitting position which calls for the strength of the torso muscles. Lean far forward (touch your toes if possible as you swing past) and drop to the other side. That forward lean stretches the back and hamstring muscles and strengthens the abdominals. Do eight side drops.

B. Seat Lift

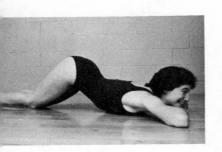

The seat lift is not really difficult, but you want to be sure you have no hidden trigger points in the lower back or groin that might feel strain. Lie prone and pretend that your chest (and only your chest) is glued to the floor. Lift your seat in the air, hold for three counts and then lower. Alternate with the gluteal and abdominal set (the third in the limbering series on page 38) six times.

B. Pelvic Tilt on the Knees

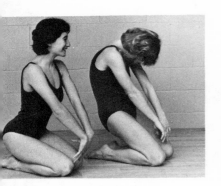

Get down on your knees and sit right down on your heels. Press your ankles flat on the floor. You can't? There are a couple of steel tendons in your ankles that won't let you. And your feet hurt? Turn to the section Relief for Hurting Feet in Chapter 7, and do the foot-limbering series daily. If you are an athlete your performance will be markedly improved. Check also to see if you have a long second toe causing that tension. Then read the section The Classic Greek Foot in Chapter 6. In the meantime wrap a small towel into a roll and put it under your ankles for support.

At the start of the exercise arch your back and press your seat out back. Then, without raising your head level more than a couple of inches, bring your seat under and pelvis forward. Return to the first position and do four.

A. Side Bend Stretch

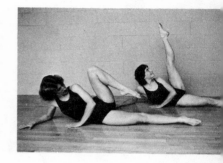

Rest on your right side. Make sure you really are on your side and not lolling back on your hip. Stretch your body out straight and point your toes. Rest your upper body on your right elbow.

Bring the left knee behind the left shoulder and keep it as close to the shoulder as you can, then straighten the leg upward. Bend the knee again and stretch it back to the starting position. Do four on each side for a set. Do four sets.

B. Hip Rotation, Sitting

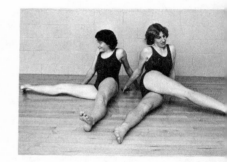

Sit, leaning back and resting on either hands or elbows. Cross the right leg over the left, twisting the leg inward until the big toe touches the floor. Stay there! Keep the leg at the same position but rotate the foot outward so that the big toe points to the ceiling. Then carry the leg back to a spread leg position and try to touch the little toe to the floor. Hold the leg open and rotate the foot inward until the toes point to the ceiling, and repeat. Alternate four times to make a set; do three sets. This reduces and strengthens thighs, and increases the range of both hip and ankle joints. If there is pain in the thighs or groin, check the adductors for trigger points.

C. Leg Extensions, Sitting

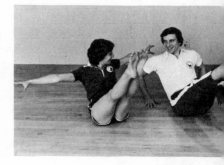

Lean back on your hands with fingers pointed forward and knees bent. Extend the right leg and then change, alternating with the left leg eight times. Then sit up and extend the arms to the sides. Repeat the alternating leg extension with bent knees but without hand support.

After you have improved, extend both arms and legs at the same time and hold for gradually increasing periods of time, starting with three seconds. This exercise provides abdominal and leg strength as well as balance.

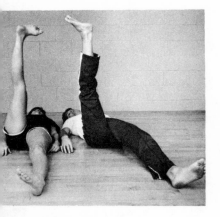

B. Supine Hip Rotation

Lie relaxed on your back and rotate the right foot outward as far as possible. Hold the foot in this position and raise the leg until it is at right angles to your body. At the peak of the lift, rotate the foot all the way in. Hold the foot rotated inward and lower the leg. Do not relax either foot or leg as you lower, merely touch the floor, and keeping the inward rotation, raise the leg overhead again. At the peak of the lift rotate the foot outward. Lower the leg in the outward position to the floor. Alternate legs doing four lifts on each side. This is excellent for strengthening leg, abdominal, lower back, and hip muscles. It, like the hip rotation, sitting exercise, will reduce thighs.

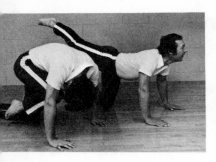

A. Knee-to-Nose Kick

Get down on all fours and bring the right knee as close to your nose as you can. Then stretch the leg back and up, at the same time raising your head. Try not to bend your arms at any time. Do eight to each side four times. This exercise stretches and strengthens the back muscles and the abdominals.

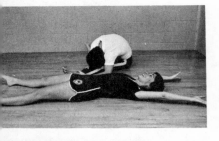

B. Roll-out and Jackknife

Lie supine with legs spread wide and arms overhead. Stretch as long as possible. Throw your upper body upward as if about to throw a basketball across the room, and with knees held straight, bring your forehead toward your left knee. Roll back down and then repeat to the right. Alternate in this manner for eight roll-outs. The abdominals are strengthened as you roll up and down. The back and hamstrings are stretched on the lean forward. The shoulders and arms are stretched on the roll-out.

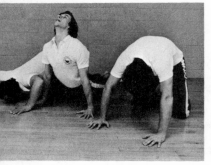

D. Peanut Push

Start on hands and knees with insteps flat on the floor. Sit back until the seat is as close to the heels as possible, the arms outstretched, the chest pressed down between spread knees. This position stretches insteps and chest and arms. Keeping the chin close to the floor, as though you were about to push a peanut across the floor with your chin, press the upper body forward. When your thighs are flat to the floor, straighten your arms and throw your head back. Then, arch your back like an angry cat, letting your head drop down while pulling your abdominals in, hard. Return to the starting position. Do six.

When you were thrusting forward "pushing the peanut," you were strengthening your arms, chest, and upper back muscles. The extended position stretched your abdominals and groin and the muscles in the front of the thighs. The humped position stretched the back and strengthened the abdominals. Altogether a difficult and valuable exercise.

C. Three Bicycles

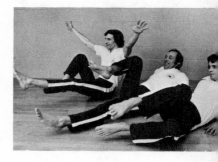

Lie supine resting on your elbows. Do a slow bicycle action with both legs for eight counts. Then, keeping both elbows in contact with the floor, roll the lower body over onto the left hip. This will work both hips and waistline. Do eight bicycle actions in this position and then alternate by doing eight to the right. Do three sets.

When you have improved considerably, try the no-hand bike the same way. Eight center, eight right, and eight left.

C. Back Leg Swing

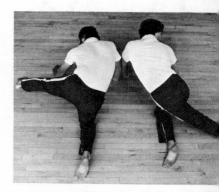

Start on all fours and carry the left leg across in back of the right foot and set the ball of the foot firmly on the floor. Keeping the leg absolutely straight, swing it around and place the foot flat on the floor in front of the left hand. Do four complete swings and then four with the other foot. That makes up a set. Do three sets. (Be sure to follow your foot with your eyes wherever it goes. This forces your back to twist.) This exercise strengthens the whole body and stretches both legs and back. The waist also come in for action as do the hips.

D. Hydrant

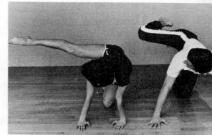

Start on all fours and raise the right leg to the side, keeping the knee bent. Then stretch the leg straight out to the side. Don't change the position or level of the upper leg at all but bend the knee again. To rest the muscles, carry the leg straight back, then repeat the hydrant. Do two to each side and work up to eight.

The hydrant works the sides of the hips we call the "saddle bags," those unsightly bumps so hard to reduce. It strengthens the lower back and gluteals and stretches the gluteus medius and the leg muscles.

C. Leg Walk-up

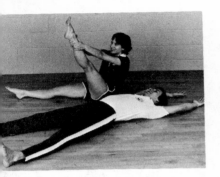

Lie supine with arms outstretched and raise one leg overhead. Swing up to grasp the leg with either or both hands and walk the hands up one over the other to the foot. The swing-up strengthens the abdominals; the walk-up stretches the back and hamstrings. Roll back down leaving the leg in the erect position. Do four with each leg.

As you improve, try to grasp higher and higher on the leg until you can reach the ankle on the first swing with no intermediate steps.

C. Push-ups—or Let-downs As the Case May Be

Another myth (of which we have a plethora in America) is that girls can't do push-ups because "they are built funny." Not so. They've simply had no training.

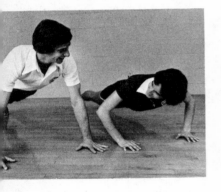

Start prone on the floor with hands flat just outside the shoulders. Keeping the body absolutely rigid, press up into a straight-arm push-up. From the top of the push-up, let yourself slowly down to the floor. Rest the arms by bringing them back along side the waist. Repeat only as long as you can maintain absolute rigidity in the back. There must be no dip or sag.

If you cannot do even one correct push-up, do a let-down. Assume the top of the push-up position with legs spread wide. Let yourself down slowly, counting to five. Get back up any way you can. When you can do five slow let-downs you will be able to do one correct push-up. When you can do three of those, bring your legs together and start with let-downs until you can do five. From then on do both.

C. Opposing Prone Arm-and-Leg Lifts

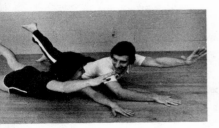

Lie prone with legs straight and arms stretched straight ahead. Raise the right arm and the left leg at the same time, and lower. Raise the left arm and the right leg simultaneously and lower. Alternate in this way eight times, and then curl into a ball to stretch the back.

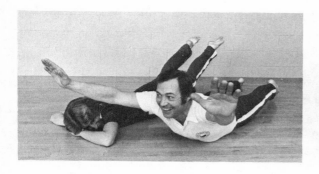
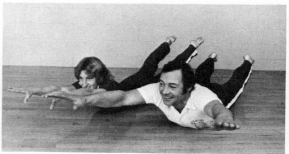

D. Prone Double Arm-and-Leg Lifts

Lie prone and lift both arms at the same time; lower. Do eight. Next, lift both legs at the same time and then lower. Do eight. Next, lift both arms and both legs at the same time; lower. Do eight. Note: This exercise is labeled *D*.

D. Rotated Bent-Knee Sit-up

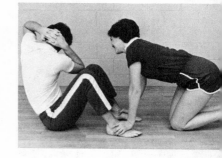

This one is not easy. One partner lies on the floor with the knees bent and feet placed fairly well apart and hands clasped behind the head. The other kneels in front and applies pressure to both ankles as an anchor. Roll over onto the left shoulder and maintain the twisted attitude as the upper body is lifted toward the sit-up position. The right elbow will be leading. Slide it outside the left knee. Maintain the same twist during the roll back down to rest on the floor. Roll then onto the other shoulder and repeat. Start with four and work to ten.

This exercise works the abdominals and virtually all the muscles in the front and sides of the torso. It is an athlete's exercise—and a dancer's.

C. Sit-up to Shoulder—Touch

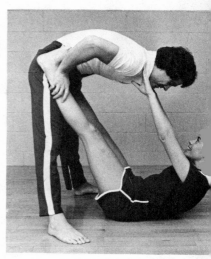

One partner lies on the floor, arms overhead and feet held at the other partner's waist. The standing partner leans forward, placing some pressure on the lying partner's feet. As the lying partner flings the arms forward and reaches up, the standing partner, with legs straight, leans forward and down. The object is to have the reaching partner touch both hands to the leaning partner's shoulders and then drop back. On the second reach the right hand crosses over to touch the standing partner's right shoulder. On the third the left hand crosses to touch the left shoulder. These three touches make up a set. Start with one set and work up to four. The exercise is for abdominal strength and hamstring stretch and is quite advanced.

Stretch Exercises

We now get into the stretch section of the program. All stretching to this point has been mild, and even those were done after plenty of warm-up. Serious stretching can *only* be done with warm muscles.

A. Stretch-outs

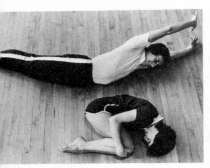

Lie on your left side and draw your knees up to your chest into the "fetal position." Then, still on your side, extend both arms straight overhead and both legs straight down. Continuing the same stretching, swinging movement, roll to the other side and collapse into the "fetal position." Four to each side will serve both to stretch and strengthen the abominals and to relax the whole body.

A. Thread Needle, Kneeling

Start on hands and knees and swing the right hand overhead. Bring it down through the space between the left hand and the knees. Try to put your shoulder and ear on the floor. Do eight with each arm. This exercise develops flexibility of the shoulders, waist, entire torso, chest, neck, and arms.

C. Thread Needle, Standing

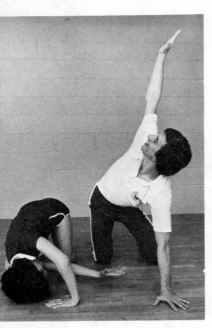

Do this exercise exactly as you did the thread needle kneeling. The only difference is that now you are standing with straight, wide-spread legs. As it is more difficult, you should start with fewer. Start with four and work up to eight on each side.

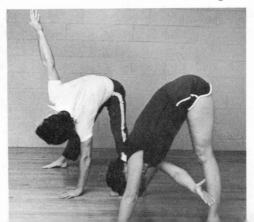

B. Hamstring Stretch, Sitting

Without flexible hamstrings, athletes are easily injured, which explains why so many of them are. Don't you be among them.

Sit spread-legged on the floor and grasp the right leg at the ankle and just below the knee. Keeping the head up, the back flat, and the legs straight, try to pull the chest down to the thigh in short easy bounces. Bounce eight times to the right and then eight to the left. Next, turn your head to the left and pull your right ear down to touch your right leg. Bounce eight right and eight left. Then grasp your ankles, one in each hand, and try to pull the chest toward the floor in eight easy bounces. Keep the head up. Finish with eight bounces with head down. Do this set three times.

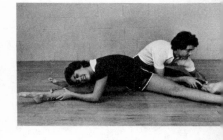

B. Heel Pull

Lie on the left side resting on your elbow. Bend your right hand *inside* the right leg and (if possible) under the right heel. If you are not flexible enough for that, grasp the lower leg where you can, but remember where you start out. As you improve you will want to appreciate your progress. Holding the right foot, straighten the leg. Do this stretch four times on the right and then four on the left. Do two sets. This stretches the arms and legs and gluteals.

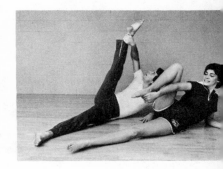

C. Prone Leg Cross-over

Lie prone with arms stretched out to the sides. Spread legs wide. Lift the right leg up from the hip without bending the knee or moving the hands from their places on the floor. When the leg is at its peak lift, bend the knee and try to bring the right foot to touch the left hand. Replace the right leg into the spread-leg position and do the exercise with the left leg. Start with three to a side and work up to six.

This exercise builds strength in the lower back and gluteals and stretches the muscles of the torso, the groin, and the fronts of the upper legs, the quads.

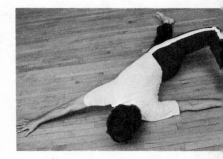

C. Stretch-outs

Start by standing with feet apart. Bend over from the hips, and keeping the knees straight, lean forward and place the hands on

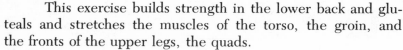

215

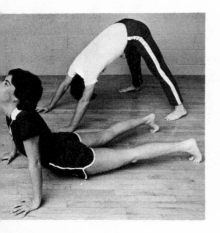

the floor. Walk your body out on your hands to the stretched-out position. Then, with your feet facing straight forward, press your heels flat on the floor and at the same time press your head down between your shoulders as though you were trying to rest your chin on your chest. From that position thrust your weight forward again onto your arms in the stretched out position as your heels leave the floor. Do this four times at the start and work up to eight.

This exercise stretches the hamstrings, especially in the lower legs. It also stretches the abdominals and groin and the fronts of the thighs. The upper back is also stretched, as both arms and chest are strengthened.

C. Seesaw

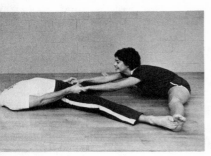

Sit opposite each other with your legs spread wide. If the flexibility and the leg length of both partners are comparable, they can each rest their feet against the other's. If one is less flexible or has shorter legs, he or she rests the feet against the other's calves. Lean forward and grasp each other's hands. Pull is exerted when one leans backward slowly and carefully at first. The one being pulled concentrates on letting go, relaxing the tight spots. Muscles will give up tension only when they are relaxed, so be careful not to overpull, which causes the reverse of what you want—tightening. Alternate for eight.

Variation on the Seesaw: The Circle

Still in the same position as before, one partner pulls back, but instead of returning to the straight sitting position, both lean to the same side—circling around as the other leans back and both move to the other side. Circle four times one way and then the other. This works hamstrings and lower back.

RELAX

Muscles need to be relaxed and rested as part of their regimen for painfree health. They can best be relaxed consciously after they have been worked vigorously. Do your exercises and then do your relaxation. Some people like to relax in silence. Others do their best when music plays. It's up to you.

A single record of a popular piece of music runs about two and a half to three minutes, so put on some slow, relaxing music and let the music slow you. Those three minutes could not be put to better use. Or get my record *Keep Fit—Be Happy*, Vol. I. On it there are two bands of relaxation to music. (See the Sources section for details.)

Tailor Rest

Sit cross-legged and allow the upper body to droop forward. Relax each segment of your body consciously starting with your head and working down neck, shoulders, arms, wrists, hands, back, legs, and feet. Sit this way for about 30 seconds (that's longer than you think).

Supine Rest

Lie back with arms and legs outstretched. If your back is very tired or stiff, bend one knee. Go through the same conscious relaxation of each part of your body. Take 30 or 40 seconds for the rundown.

Side Rest

Roll over onto your side and again go through the complete relaxation rundown.

Prone Rest

Roll over into the prone position and draw up one leg as in the illustration on page 146. This is a wonderful back rester. Go through the relaxation rundown in this position.

ONE LAST REMINDER

If you want to get the most from your exercise program you have to enjoy it. Music is one of the best aids; good companions are another. Noticing improvement is a third, and measurements can help there. You might overlook the fact that you no longer puff on the stairs, but you'll be sure to spot your slimming waistline. Be more aware of yourself and what happens to you each day. If your sex life improves, exercise may be helping. If your golf handicap is dropping, don't just give exercise some credit—double your exercise time.

Myotherapy can make you painfree, but it is the exercise that will keep you that way. Remember these basics.

1. Make a history of yourself that may give you clues as to *why* you hurt *where* you hurt.
2. Search out and erase trigger points wherever they are hiding.
3. Stretch the muscles involved and bring them to their full, resting, painfree length.
4. Get into shape and stay that way with a fitness program suitable for *you*.
5. Observe the emotional climate you live in. If it is destructive, change it.

My Blessings

There is nothing new under the sun—or moon either for that matter. Everything was always here in one form or another. Dr. Travell says myotherapy was born of serendipity. Dr. Tivy says it came about because known facts were seen from a different angle—without the limitations imposed by long training in one field to the exclusion of knowledge in most others.

Whatever the elements gathered during its gestation, whatever or whoever is responsible for its birth, myotherapy is here now, for you to use.

Use it in good health.

218

Afterword

IN DEFENSE OF BONNIE PRUDDEN
by Dr. Desmond R. Tivy

As a physician, one can't help wondering about the advisability of publishing medical discoveries directly to the lay public. My own ethos would not lead me to do it that way. Medical discoveries are normally published first in the medical literature, step by tedious step, for exposure to harsh peer criticism. That which can readily be refuted is probably false; that which the many can find little fault with is probably true; and many shades of grey exist between the two. Only rarely is a lifetime's work exposed to view all at once, and when it is, oftentimes others have independently discovered and published most of it already. (A noted cousin of mine, some seven generations back, Isaac Newton, nearly suffered this fate.)

To publish in the medical literature requires (1) the possession of a medical or scientific degree, and usually and preferably a position and reputation of some standing; (2) painstaking record keeping of results, with control normals to compare them with; (3) usually and preferably severe limitation of interest to selected portions of results that can be studied independently of extraneous factors; (4) the spending of considerable time learning the entire output of others in the field; and (5) learning the proper methods of research. Bonnie Prudden has none of these requirements, except that her record keeping is reasonably good for an amateur. I have only the medical degree, and didn't even do the work itself about which she has written.

My approach would be to attempt to involve others, who have the necessary qualifications, in the research and publication process. In my own small way I have attempted to do this, but I find it an uphill task, with little time, between the de-

219

mands of a busy medical practice and of my family, in which to pursue it. Others have attempted to sell inadequately tested medical ideas directly to the lay public. Doctors naturally resent this, and it prejudices them against such ideas, which is the main reason why I would not have published this book.

But Bonnie Prudden is no longer young (except at heart and in demeanor), and she is not prepared to await the slow process of medical acceptance and dissemination until after she has been long dead. And I have indeed noticed that publication of medical ideas in the lay press seems to be the quickest way of being shot down if you are wrong, and of stimulating competent research if you are right. (A noted authority on cholesterol, oft published in prestigious medical journals, affirmed to me that the acceptance of his somewhat unpopular ideas, which I feel will turn out to be largely correct, goes up by quantum leaps every time they hit *The New York Times*, but seem to be shelved, ostrich-like, after each *medical* publication, even though his peers could find little fault with his argument.) So I wish her all good luck with her endeavor; and my comments are an attempt to forestall some of the criticism and prejudice that she will receive by publication.

You may wonder how it is that I feel competent to judge her work. I have practiced medicine for nearly 30 years; my surgical residency years included a good deal of orthopedic training; my ego has always been better satisfied with attacking unsolved problems, than memorizing the solution to solved problems (for once solved they become too easy and too many others can do it as well or better); I have studied something of the history of science, and of epistemology, and find both entirely fascinating; I have been brought up to question revealed wisdom very critically, and so I have never really believed that those patients, whose pain my profession could not explain or cure, were the victims of an overzealous imagination, or neurotic, or psychologically sick, or whatever (at least not nearly as often as my teachers would have me think); I have been in general practice for the last 13 years, with the luxury to pick and choose, among a wide range of human ills, to treat those in which I had the greatest insight, and to refer the rest to others; performing only the most minor of surgery these days, I have tried to enlarge on non-operative ways to deal with musculo-skeletal pain; and I have, as stated in the Foreword, referred several hundreds of patients to Bonnie Prudden for treatment of most of the conditions she writes about.

I have found that her success rate, in those cases that I have referred to her (as well as in some that were referred by others), has been far higher than anything I could achieve by orthodox medical therapy, no matter what conventional expertise I call in for help. Or else, she tends to produce results more speedily, less painfully, more safely, and/or at less cost than my profession could have done. So successful has been the prolonged relief of symptoms (notice I didn't say "cure"—*nothing* is ever cured, unless you take it out, or you develop a vaccine for it, or you're dead!)—so successful, that when it doesn't work as expected, a reappraisal of the initial diagnosis, by further testing, usually shows that the diagnosis was wrong.

In essence, myotherapy works on, and only on, disorders of function. The medical profession is good at treating disorders of structure, but has always been weak on function. Myotherapy cannot influence structure. The distinction between function and structure may seem clear enough, but I must admit that the two tend to become blurred at the sub-microscopic level.

Thus what myotherapy seems able to do, the doctors tend to be weak at. And what the doctors are good at, myotherapy can't help. What a superb complementation of one with the other! Here is a perfect opportunity for the medical profession to increase its success rate, and here is Bonnie Prudden offering it to us on a plate!

But does it really *work*? And on exactly what kinds of pain? Could Bonnie Prudden, and could I, with all our attempts at honest self-criticism, be deluding ourselves? Yes, it's remotely possible, of course, which is why what she has found, and what I have found, is as naught until confirmed (or, heaven forbid, disproved) by repeated medical testing and research by many people in many places quite independently. Only then will we "know." What is probable is that others will be able to confirm *most* of our results (discarding the fallacious), and *add* some results we had not yet discovered.

But haven't the world's researchers better things to do than spend their restricted time and funds looking into every crank and crackpot idea that someone has dreamed up? Shouldn't the originator of the novel idea be the one to present it, in finished form, to the world for peer review and expert criticism? The answer to both questions is, of course, "Yes, in most cases."

But there is another side to the coin. In the first place, this is a very important subject, involving extremely common forms of human pain, not just a piece of intellectual trivia. Even if the qualified reader has not happened to find that at least some of the things put forward in this book gel with his experience, then it doesn't take much time and effort to mount a limited trial on just a few people. The more it works on the few, the more it becomes worth it to extend the trial to the many. The enormous potential reward seems to merit a very modest gamble.

Secondly, Bonnie Prudden has here presented the evidence in as finished a form as she is capable of presenting. Her approach has been as scientific as she is trained to be. Had she possessed a degree in medicine or physical therapy, she could have known how to do it better, but had she spent time to acquire such, she would then have had to unlearn some of it too, and she would have been too blinded to see what she has seen. And it doesn't become real evidence until what she has noted is confirmed by others of repute.

Usually, when laymen take on the experts, they fail to take the precaution to examine the known facts (evidence) first, or at least only learn a small and insufficient portion of them. Velikovsky was a typical example of this, and Carl Sagan, with superiority in volume of data, demolished him with extraordinary fairness and patience (*Broca's Brain*, Chapter 7). But Bonnie Prudden is working in an area where there are many theories but little data. All she is doing here is presenting some more preliminary data; let the theoreticians do what they will with it. If some theoreticians choose to believe that what she says is impossible, then let them go out and try it, and if they can confirm her results, then reexamine their theories and choose which ones to discard as no longer consistent with the data; and if they choose to call her approach unscientific, then let them read Carl Sagan (*Broca's Brain*, Chapter 2) for a superb five-page discourse on the scientific method, as exciting in a literary sense, as in an intellectual one. They will thus be reminded that data do not become impossible because they do not fit entrenched theories—it becomes the other way around! The key to all this, of course, is the validation of the observed data, and that is what is called for as the next chapter in the myotherapy story. But theory? That comes later.

Theories are useful as predictors of future data: the better they predict, the better they are (and conversely). They are also extremely useful as a conceptual "handle" to hold on to while thinking about a subject, and while discussing it with others. I have urged Bonnie Prudden not to get into this aspect of her work, since whatever she, or I, theorize will probably turn out to be wrong, and it would be a pity to be judged by one's mistakes, the baby being thrown out with the bath water.

But it really is extraordinarily difficult to discuss such a subject *without* bringing in theoretical constructs, or at least very clumsy. Have you ever thought about how difficult it would be to "explain" a television set to a fourteenth-century audience? The centuries of preliminary step taking and concept building would have to be compressed beyond the limits of comprehension. The gaps in the chain of reasoning of "from the familiar to the unknown" are just too great.

So it is here: We do not have a valid understanding of what pain is. We can understand why pain may run from B to A, but not why it also seems to run from C to A, or even A to C. If we bruise a bone, it is quite easy to form a mental picture of the cellular, biochemical, and neuronal steps that give rise to the resultant pain in that bone; but if a pain arises there without injury, and without evidence of other structural change, it is difficult to comprehend what is happening, especially if the pain is referred to another area without shared nerve pathway. One is then forced to postulate other pathways—but what other?

One can speculate like mad, as those working on acupuncture, biofeedback, and the like have done, on the possible role of the recently "in" subject of endorphins, and of neurovascular and neuromuscular pathways, and of bio-electric-potential pathways, and about electronic negative feedback, and so forth. One can theorize about psychological mechanisms too, but this only dodges the issue of how *they* might work. Once again, we need more data, and the theory can follow.

So far, I have, for reasons of difficulty, deliberately avoided discussion of what types of pain I tend to refer for myotherapy. Where history or physical findings suggest structural disease, such as nerve impingement, tumor, or arthritic inflammation, for instance, then of course I use the normal medical or surgical approach. But where such is *not* suggested, thus suggesting a disorder of function (and I *don't* mean a "functional disorder" in the pejorative sense of a neurotic, psychological, one), I think of myotherapy as a possible simplest answer to the problem. For, when all is said and done, it is really simplicity that we seek. Any fool can reach a complicated solution. (I suppose my hobby of recreational mathematics has led me to think that way—or perhaps it's the other way around!)

Simplicity and safety, however, do not always go together. In fact, they are often inversely proportional to one another, thus demanding a compromise between the two. It is of course much safer, from the point of view of subsequent criticism, to use an accepted modality that only sometimes works, than an experimental method that usually works, especially if you are tempted to use it when it might be inappropriate. But if you start, as I did, with those cases that have been exhaustively studied for structural disease, with negative results, or with those patients that refuse to be so studied, then you are on safer ground. But after you have found, as I did, some gratifying results, when is it reasonable to take shortcuts in the diagnostic process?

The purist will of course say "never," without consideration of the cost in time, money, and discomfort, not to mention possible dangers in the testing process itself (such as inordinate exposure to X-rays); his reputation for thoroughness is at stake. To be "sure," rather than intelligently guess a bit, is an expensive luxury, however, and the medical profession, in trying to do just that, is pricing itself out of the public reach. Thus, in striving for simplicity, in cutting of costs (in all three above-mentioned meanings of the word), I now feel comfortable to try myotherapy on selected cases, when the probability of the presence of organic disease is low, without first testing exhaustively, but not (yet!) without an appraisal of the problem to a lesser or greater degree. At some later time, I may feel able to verbalize what parameters I choose to guide me in such a choice, but for the moment I will stick to the above generalizations. Others may be able to take up the task, too.

On the subject of safety, one should consider the known side effects of myotherapy. In my experience, they comprise the following, *and no other:*

1. *Pain.* The treatment by pressure hurts for a few seconds, commensurate with the pain of an intramuscular injection

of a mildly irritant substance, but often less than the pain involved in injecting saline or local anesthetic into exactly the same tender spot (trigger point). It certainly seems less than the pain of injecting around an inflamed tendon, as in "bursitis" of the shoulder.

2. *Bruising.* Bruises at the site of pressure do sometimes occur. They are very small in extent, and occur more often in women, who are known to bruise easily. They are less common and less extensive than would be likely to occur were the same spot injected. Those on anti-coagulants will bruise more readily, of course. Our experience with such patients is limited, but it has so far not been a problem.

3. *Increased function leading to careless behavior.* A few have celebrated their new-found mobility and freedom from pain by going dancing or engaging in some other activity inappropriate to their degree of control, thus ending up falling and doing themselves harm. (I am not being entirely facetious if I call this a side effect, rather than a therapeutic triumph.)

4. *Pain shift.* A unilateral pain may switch sides after treatment; or it may shift from one area to another. Our experience is that, the fact that the pain can do this at all confirms the probability that the disorder is functional, not structural. Further treatment, to the new areas, usually results in further pain relief.

5. *Pain exacerbation, with or without pain shift.* Usually this means either structural disease, such as a herniated disc, which has been overlooked, or severe superimposed inflammatory reaction, and/or psychological overlay. In any of these cases, medical treatment is required. With careful selection of cases, this is rare in our experience.

6. *Temporary relief—no lasting benefit.* Here the diagnosis may be wrong, or there is more than one diagnosis; or the patient is improperly motivated (for a multitude of possible reasons) to continue exercises and other home treatment to prevent recurrences; or occasionally, for undetermined reasons.

7. *Dollar cost.* Though the Prudden Institute of Myotherapy's charges per hour are equal to or slightly less than the going rate for physical therapy, the number of sessions required is usually far less than that incurred with physical therapy (or, for that matter, chiropractic), so the total cost is less. And if, by taking a gamble, expensive testing is also obviated, then the cost

is often less than the testing process itself. But at present, the absence of third-party insurance coverage for myotherapy does deter a significant number of people from the initial cost. (There is no reason why, if more myotherapists are trained, with no training costs themselves to absorb, the cost of myotherapy should not drop significantly.)

8. *If the indication to use it is wrong, it won't work!* This applies to almost everything, of course.

Now at first glance, this may seem quite a list. But the more you think about it, and think about the comparable lists that you would have to honestly draw up in assessing alternative approaches to the pain problem, the more innocuous my list becomes. For instance, if aspirin had to have the informational package insert that prescription drugs must have, it is very doubtful that the F.D.A. would approve it, let alone anyone dare swallow a tablet. And yet we all (except those allergic or otherwise intolerant) happily dose ourselves with it without a thought, because it is *relatively* safe.

So it is with myotherapy. I find that the benefit/side-effect ratio of myotherapy is one of the highest of any treatment I have available to me in the practice of medicine. I wish it worked on other diseases too! It all hangs on the question of *diagnosis*. If your treatment is dangerous, you had better get the right diagnosis, no matter the cost, before you embark on it. If your treatment is safe, you can sometimes afford to guess a bit, and see what happens. How else did the old saw, "Take two aspirins, and call me in the morning," become current? And if you are damn fool enough to take two aspirins for a crushing pain in the front of your 40-year-old chest, then God help you (and He may not!), and then I suppose you might try myotherapy instead—though you won't find Bonnie Prudden or any of her trainees will agree to do it; they know better. And it could be doubly foolish to try it, if you could find somebody foolhardy enough to go along with you, because your pain might temporarily go away, leading you to a false sense of reassurance; but, as with nitroglycerin, it won't *stay* away, which should tell you something, and direct your steps to the hospital, where you belong.

It is sad that the exact diagnosis, in many cases of pain, is sometimes so hard to come by—else side effect number 8 would never apply. Bonnie Prudden and her staff therapists make it a rule never to treat patients unless they have cleared the visit with a doctor first. This, for the moment at least, is as it should be. For it is, at present, an experimental therapy, whose list of side effects has not yet been substantiated by independent observers, performed by persons not trained in medical diagnosis (they could be trained some, but that would be the more dangerous, for then they might *think* they knew). The only exception to the "doctor-referred only" rule seems to be that, when Bonnie is lecturing on the subject, a volunteer is often brought forward to have his pain "fixed." One does not expect that such volunteers really think that a diagnosis has been offered, but rather that they can maybe cancel that trip to the psychiatrist, after all, since the doctor seems to have been wrong when he told them that the pain was "all in their head."

But *was* he wrong? Maybe, indeed probably, most of it *is* in their head, but not quite in the pejorative way that all too many doctors half-sneeringly imply. A psychiatrist could spend years trying to erase the pain (in your head) of your toothache; even if and when he succeeded, a dentist could, by extraction, have corrected the problem considerably earlier! If the pain you incur after repeated falls to the left on the ski slope cannot be corrected by a visit to the left-ski repairman, don't let anyone tell you that your problem resides in the head! It *does* reside there, but no psychiatrist can remedy the matter. The problem is that your head is telling your legs and body the wrong way to turn left, so go see a ski instructor! Thus if the muscles in the left side of your back are hurting, and competent doctors can't find anything "wrong" with your back, maybe the problem is neither structural nor psychosomatic, but a functional problem, and the simplest approach may be to visit a myotherapist.

But do the doctors themselves, and the physical therapists they call in to assist them, not also treat functional musculo-skeletal problems? Yes, of course they do, and until I came across Bonnie Prudden, I used the same techniques they do, and to this day I still use them, when it seems appropriate. But my willingness to try something new is only sustained if the results so obtained are superior to the old ways of doing it. My enthusiasm for myotherapy exists because I find it *works*, and works, in general, more quickly, more effectively, more predictably, often less expensively, and just as, or more, safely, than its conventional alternatives.

227

If Bonnie Prudden has done nothing else for me, she has enabled me to develop a better conceptual understanding of some of the types of pain in which myotherapy can be so successful, and of the common ground between the successes and failures of orthodox and unorthodox treatments for such pain. For instance, acupuncture went through quite a vogue a few years back (though I never had my patients use it), and then public interest died down. Why? It would appear that it often relieved pain, after innumerable treatments, and after enormous expense, but seldom lastingly. I begin to see why relief was temporary, for if acupuncture relieves the same kind of pain that myotherapy does (and maybe the frequent coincidence of acupuncture points and trigger points is more than coincidental), then unless you treat the cause of the pain, it will return. And if the cause be, for instance, muscle function related to posture, unless you "teach" the muscles better subsequent habits, the cycle will start all over again.

Myotherapy, however, does not pretend to influence internal organs, as, I believe, acupuncturists claim to do. But I can now understand why they thought they could. I have seen a number of cases of abdominal pain, for instance, that patients were persuaded were due to gall bladder disease, and the patient could not understand why the X-rays were always negative. After myotherapy, and pain relief for a year and more (whereas previous pains occurred almost every week, which is unlikely periodicity for gall bladder disease anyway), it seems to me the pain was musculo-skeletal in the first place, secondary to postural deficits. But I can quite understand that the patient and her therapist might imagine that it was her gall bladder that had been "cured."

As another example, I think I now understand why Kurland's acupressure only sometimes works on cases of migraine. He advocates the same sort of pressure used in myotherapy, on only four of the trigger points that are used by myotherapists, and subsequent exercises are not stressed. If only *part* of the full treatment is used, no wonder it fails in some cases! This too is a trap for the unwary reader of this book. Anyone who tries myotherapy, and doesn't do it right, can expect failure, as can anyone who takes only one penicillin tablet to rid himself of a sore throat. It is remarkable that children can be quickly taught how to use myotherapy on their parents with quite good results,

228

provided the areas needing attention do not change. When they do change, they would need to return to the trained myo-therapist for another lesson.

And I think I now understand, for the same reasons as given regarding acupressure, why standard physical therapy works and fails when it does, though its results tend to be longer lasting than acupressure, because attention is given to future preventive measures. And why transcutaneous electrical nerve stimulation, and biofeedback (both very time-consuming and expensive), succeed and fail when they do, for analogous reasons. And certainly why proponents of multiple injections into trigger points only sometimes succeed: You just cannot treat a few trigger points, and do nothing about the rest—it just doesn't work. To my mind, Bonnie Prudden's great and key contribution here has been the discovery of in just how many unexpected places trigger points may lurk.

And what of chiropractic? I know little of their work and methods, but the anecdotal evidence of good results is just too overwhelming to ignore. The overtones of the word *manipulation* do conjure up the image of possible dangers that myo-therapy could never encounter. But I must say that if the medical profession could produce as relatively few disasters as one hears from the chiropractors, I would be the more ready to criticize the methods of the latter. Even if there were twice the rate of incompetence among chiropractors as among doctors (for which I have no supposition or evidence), their "toys" seem a lot less dangerous to play with than some of ours!

It would seem entirely possible that myotherapy and chiropractic succeed on the same types of pain, via different approaches, possibly via similar mechanisms. But several important differences arise. First, chiropractic is a passive therapy, which the therapist does on you while you lie back. Little attempt is made to prepare the way against recurrent pain, so you return week after week for a dose of the same medicine. Myo-therapy, at least as practiced by Bonnie Prudden, though passive at start, demands continued patient effort to reeducate the patient into non-pain-producing habits. The necessity for multiple visits would be deemed a failure of the method, or of the therapist, or of the patient's resolve. As a rough rule, I find that it takes about as many visits to the myotherapist, to ensure full pain relief, as the first figure of one's age. This reflects the concept that pain erasure seems to be an unlearning process (followed by relearning), and that children have less to forget than their elders, and learn faster afterward. Subsequent repeat visits are required when time, new bad postural habits, or new injuries supervene. But some patients, apparently unweanable from passivity, will still prefer the chiropractic approach. And I must admit that the Flock does seem to behave better if a visit to the Pastor is required at regular intervals.

Another important difference between chiropractic and myotherapy is that the latter makes no claim to treat internal diseases, which claims are the least substantiated of the chiropractors' results. A possible exception is the case of those conditions thought to be structural and internal (such as hemorrhoids) where in reality all that is complained of is pain in the same region, which is not the same thing at all.

Another difference is that myotherapists are (insofar as I can influence them) under no illusions that they are treating the spine and its nerves, and do not hypothesize unsubstantiatable theories about their work. I have always thought that if chiropractors would keep quiet about their theories, the doctors might listen to them more. But I wish I and my colleagues were blameless in this respect. I understand *why* they theorize; it has its uses, but it is counterproductive at present.

The final difference between chiropractors and myotherapists is that the former take X-rays and claim to diagnose, the latter do not. This upsets the doctors more than anything else, as we feel we have the best training around in diagnosis, and this is really indisputable. A properly trained myotherapist will not treat a case not checked by a physician (or in the case of TMJ dysfunction, a dentist) and will only give an opinion as to the advisability of continued therapy versus further medical treatment after the first session.

Which brings us to a very important area, that of control. Bonnie Prudden has no aspirations to found a second quasi-medical, politically accepted empire as the chiropractors have done. Her only aspiration is to found a school of myotherapists, and see if the world can use its products. She "certifies" her therapists, when she finds them as competent as she, because there is no one else around to do it. There is no reason in the world why state governments cannot license myotherapists, as they do nurses and physical therapists (and physicians and chiropractors, too), and set up governing bodies to control standards of education and ethics. Indeed, if the idea catches on, it will have to be that way.

At present Bonnie Prudden keeps a tight rein on standards and ethics personally, so that her trainees all follow the pattern she has set. But eventually, among the nth generation of trainees, some bad apples are bound to appear, and that is what licensing is all about. Remember that the first members of all the licensed professions were unlicensed too (and when some of them became unlicensed in another sense, government stepped in). Whether government, which sees fit to let a druggist sell you an aspirin without first seeing the doctor, will ever see fit to let you see a myotherapist for a limited session or two without first seeing a doctor, remains to be seen. In an ideal world it would probably be OK, but the world is not ideal.

It is very difficult to predict which ideas will catch on. It seems to me that this one should, and probably will. But if I invent a pill that cures a certain disease 100 percent of the time (it never happens), if the patient populace finds it too bitter, and usually won't swallow it, my success rate will plummet to near zero. So patient compliance and motivation are a key part of all new (and old) medical therapies. My patients comply with myotherapy as well as or better than with other forms of treatment, but my patients, and those attracted to Bonnie Prudden referred by other doctors, are a select group, unrepresentative of the population at large. Will the populace at large fare as well as our patients? I don't see how it is possible to predict this. I expect them to, but time may tell.

A word should be said about arthritis. There are 90-odd forms of arthritis listed in the medical literature, and doubtless more to follow. Most people know about degenerative osteoarthritis, which may develop with age and after injury, and which shows up on X-rays. And they usually know about the inflammatory types of arthritis, such as rheumatoid arthritis and LE (lupus erythematosus) and gout, which can occur in younger patients. Of the less common types they remain in fortunate ignorance.

But one type not mentioned among the 90-odd, the commonest type of all, is the arthritis-that-isn't—the type the doctor says you have when he really means pain. My patients sometimes ask whether it is true that Bonnie Prudden "cures arthritis." No, of course not, but she does often relieve the *diagnosis* of arthritis-that-wasn't, or at least wasn't the cause of the symptoms. For if your 60-year-old painful neck is X-rayed, osteoarthritis will commonly be found, but that is not to say that the osteoarthritis is the cause of your pain. It may be, but more commonly it is setting the stage for improper muscle function, which can usually be relieved by myotherapy. And since the pain is relieved concomitantly, and the X-rays still show osteoarthritis subsequently, one can only conclude that it was the muscle dysfunction that caused the pain—which will return unless the muscles are "taught" to behave more comfortably in the future.

In similar fashion, myotherapy can achieve pain relief in a number of organic, structural diseases that are episodic in nature, with quiescent periods between flare-ups. It would seem that not all the crippling that occurs in rheumatoid arthritis, or even multiple sclerosis, is due to the disease itself (much as not all the pain associated with osteoarthritis is due to the arthritis itself). While only physicians can (or, at least, can attempt to) deal with the acute flare-ups, myotherapy can sometimes relieve the pain, probably due to disuse stiffness, that occurs in the quiet intervals. Physical therapists know this too.

I have always disliked the term *trigger point.* Apart from being inartistic, it does not convey the right message. I could suggest *myalgic points* as closer, but I am not entirely happy with that either. I am not even too happy with the word *myotherapy*, even though I coined it myself (or did I? Is anything ever original?). I am happier with *myotherapist*, conveying the impression of a therapist who not only treats pain in muscle (and its extensions in tendon, aponeurosis, and fascia) but also works to "teach" the muscle new habits afterward. But *is* the pain thus treated *in* muscle, or is it the nerve endings in or near the muscle that are the target? Who knows?

If myotherapy can be safely developed for preliminary use *before* consulting a physician, or if physicians can ever feel safe prescribing it before engaging in a series of expensive definitive diagnostic tests, then myotherapy could make a significant contribution toward solving the problem of the escalating costs of medical care.

I find myotherapy sometimes useful as a diagnostic test; I find it teachable to other therapists, and even, in limited fashion, to patients; I find it remarkably effective and largely predictable; and I find it safe. I hope the world will agree, and can use it.

July 1980
Lee, Massachusetts

232

Appendix 1
Muscle and Skeletal Plates of the Human Body

INTRODUCTION TO THE PLATES

Plates 1 and 2 are front and back views of the human skeleton. The various areas usually housing pain have been boxed and labeled with roman numerals. To find the muscles on a specific area of the body, check the following table.

Body Part	Section	Plate No.
Abdominals	XV	6
Arm	X	16, 17
Axilla (armpit) (not indicated on Plates 1 and 2)	XVI	18
Back, lower	I	5
Back, upper	II	5, 13
Chest	IX	6
Face	XIV	12, 15
Feet	VIII	11
Groin	III	6
Hand	XI	16, 17
Head	XIII	12, 13, 14, 15
Leg, lower (back)	V	8, 9, 10
Leg, lower (inner aspect)—		
Leg, lower (outer aspect)—		
Leg, lower (front)	VII	7, 9, 10
Leg, upper (back)	IV	8, 9, 10
Leg, upper (inner aspect)—		
Leg, upper (outer aspect)—		
Leg, upper (front)	VI	7, 9, 10
Neck	XII	6, 13, 14, 15
Pelvic floor or levator ani (not indicated on Plates 1 and 2)	XVII	19

Plates 3 and 4, Muscle Man, are front and back views of the whole body. These will give you an overall look at the human body, and, should you be interested, they also provide you with the names of the streets you will be traveling along.

Plate 5 contains sections I and II, the lower and upper back. On this and other plates you will see small circles, some of which are labeled with arabic numbers. They indicate the spots most likely to contain trigger points—and in the order in which our experience says they should be checked.

It is not essential, however, that you follow the number sequences as we have outlined them. These work for us, and they will be helpful to you in the beginning. In time you too will develop techniques which suit your temperament and skills.

The only numbers we have given you that are out of sequence with the work presented are spots 7 and 8 in the belt area. We suggested you apply pressure to spot 8 before spot 7. That is because it is easier to learn the pulling-in motion than the push-away.

The dotted lines between the circles are there to make it easier for you to get from one place to another along a known route. They also show you exactly where you are on the muscle hidden from you by the skin covering. It was only after we combined the trigger point work with the visual aid of anatomy charts that we began to understand what was happening. While it is not difficult to find and press on a trigger point, it is both more interesting and efficient when you know what you are doing and where you are doing it.

Also on Plate 5 you will see two "grids." The one on the left side covers the latissimus dorsi; the one on the right, the scapula (shoulder blade). Consider that every square may house a trigger point.

Plate 6, the front of the torso, covers sections III, the groin; IX, the chest; XII, the neck; and XV, the abdomen.

Plates 7, 8, 9, and 10 are all aspects of the leg, sections IV, V, VI, and VII. Please understand that when you are working on either the upper or lower leg, it is essential that both inner and outer aspects be covered as well as the front and back.

Plate 11, the feet, section VIII.

Plate 12, sections XIII and XIV, brings you the front view of the face and head. Here you meet for the first time a "line." A line merely means that you work along it from one point to another. Line A means you work along the cheekbone. Line B indicates you work from the eye to the ear.

Plate 13 brings you the back of the head, the neck, and the upper back, or shoulders—sections XIII, XII and II. Here you have a grid, a line, and the circles indicating spots that are usually sensitive.

Plate 14, the neck, side view. Sections XII and XIII.

Plate 15, the side of the head, neck, and face. Sections XIII, XII, and XIV. On this plate your "line" circles the ear.

Plates 16 and 17 show the arms and hands. Sections X and XI.

Plate 18 is of section XVI, the axilla, a very sensitive spot if there is arm or hand pain, or chest or upper back pain. It is a key spot for any who use their arms and hands either hard, as in sport, or often, as in typing.

Plate 19 shows section XVII, the pelvic floor or levator ani. This plate is provided so you can see how any injury to the coccyx or the pubic arch or pelvic bones could affect the muscles of the pelvis. Such injury could then cause such seemingly unrelated or spontaneous problems as frigidity, impotence, or pain attributed to hemorrhoids.

GUIDE TO THE LOCATION OF TRIGGER POINTS

In this list, the roman numerals refer to sections of the skeleton according to the system shown in Plates 1 and 2. The arabic numerals refer to the spots on the body that most often house trigger points and should always be checked when working on a particular body part. This list tells in which muscle each spot is found. The numbering system is used in Plate 3 through Plate 19 and in the text.

It is certainly not essential that you learn the names of these muscles, but in time you will find the names of many sticking in your mind just like the names of people you meet often or work with. It is easier to be exact in your work if you have a definite name than if you have to rely on "who-sis," "what-sis," or "hey you!"

Sections I and II: Lower and upper back

1. Gluteus maximus and medius
2. Gluteus maximus and medius
3. Gluteus maximus and medius
4. Gluteus medius
5. Gluteus medius
6. Gluteus medius

7. The "belt," aponeurosis latissimus dorsi
8. The "belt," aponeurosis latissimus dorsi
9. The "belt," external oblique
10. The "belt," external oblique
11. Latissimus dorsi

12. Teres major
13. Infraspinatus
14. Trapezius
15. Trapezius
16. Trapezius
17. Trapezius

18. Splenius capitis (lower attachment)

19. Gluteus maximus (proximity of coccyx)

Grid D: Scapula
Grid E: Latissimus dorsi

Sections III (groin), IX (chest), XII (neck), and XV (abdomen)

20. Pectoralis major
21. Pectoralis major
22. Pectoralis major
23. Pectoralis minor
24. Pectoralis below clavicle (collarbone)
25. Pectoralis above clavicle
26. Abdominals: upper attachment to the ribs
27. Inguinal line proximity of iliopsoas
28. Pubic arch at symphysis
29. Inguinal line proximity of pectineus
30. Iliac crest

Section VI: Upper leg, front
31. Tensor fasciae latae
32. Tensor fasciae latae
33. Vastus medialis
34. Vastus lateralis
35. Rectus femoris

Section IV: Upper leg, back
36. Adductor magnus and semitendinosus
37. Biceps femoris and vastus lateralis
38. Biceps femoris

Upper leg, outer aspect
39. Tensor fasciae latae and vastus lateralis
40. Tensor fasciae latae and vastus lateralis (lower)

Upper leg, inner aspect
41. Adductor magnus
42. Gracilis

Section VII: Lower leg, front
43. Anterior tibialis
44. Soleus

Section V: Lower leg, back
45. Gastrocnemius
46. Gastrocnemius
47. Soleus

Lower leg, outer aspect
48. Peroneus longus
49. Lateral malleolus

Section VIII: The foot
50. Extensor digitorum brevis
51. Extensor digitorum brevis
52. Abductor digiti minimi
53. Plantar aponeurosis
54. Abductor hallucis longus
55. Plantar region (sole)

237

Sections XIV and XII: Anterior views of face and head

60. Orbicularis oculi 1
61. Orbicularis oculi 2
62. Procerus
63. Nasalis

Grid A: Frontalis
Line A: Zygomaticus major and minor
Line B: Temporalis

Sections XII and XIII: Side of the head and face and neck

Line C: Around the ear

64. Platysma
65. Mastoid process
66. Splenius capitis
67. Sternocleidomastoid (posterior edge)
68. Sternocleidomastoid (anterior edge)
69. Squeeze technique on sternocleidomastoid
70. Trapezius
71. Trapezius
72. Trapezius
73. Sternocleidomastoid: sternum attachment
74. Sternocleidomastoid: clavicle attachment

Line B: Temporalis
Grid B: Temporalis

Sections II, XII, and XIII: Posterior view of head, neck, and upper back

Grid C
Line D

70. Trapezius, neck
71. Trapezius, neck
72. Trapezius, neck

14. Trapezius, shoulders
15. Trapezius, shoulders
16. Trapezius, shoulders
17. Trapezius, shoulders
18. Splenius capitis, lower attachment

Sections X and XI: Arms and hands
75. Brachioradialis
76. Extensor carpi radialis longus
77. Extensor digitorum
78. Extensor carpi radialis longus
79. Brachialis
80. Deltoid
81. Pronator teres
82. Flexor carpi ulnaris
83. Thenar eminence
84. Palmar aponeurosis
85. Adductor pollicis

Section XVI: Axilla
We have not provided numbers for the axilla because, like the grid areas, there are no specific spots. The entire area is suspect in regard to trigger points, and all of it needs to be checked.

Section XVII: Pelvic floor (Levator Ani)
The floor of the pelvis is numberless too. This plate is provided to show you how many muscles line the pelvis. This should remind you that damage to the back, side, front, rim, and even the interior of the pelvis can affect any of the openings passing through it, such as the anal canal. Damage can also affect neighboring structures, for example, the prostate.

PLATE 1

THE SKELETON, FRONT VIEW
Sections of the Body

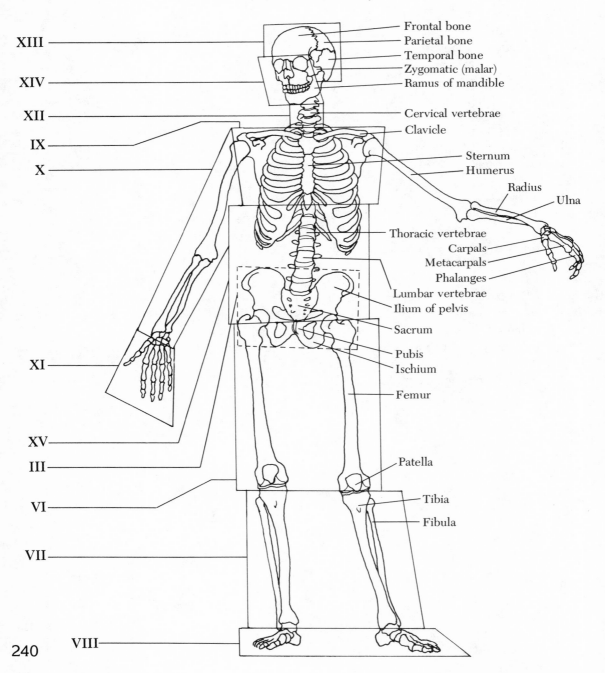

XIII

XIV

XII

IX

X

XI

XV

III

VI

VII

240 VIII

Frontal bone
Parietal bone
Temporal bone
Zygomatic (malar)
Ramus of mandible

Cervical vertebrae

Clavicle

Sternum
Humerus
Radius
Ulna

Thoracic vertebrae
Carpals
Metacarpals
Phalanges

Lumbar vertebrae
Ilium of pelvis

Sacrum

Pubis
Ischium

Femur

Patella

Tibia

Fibula

PLATE 2

THE SKELETON, BACK VIEW
Sections of the Body

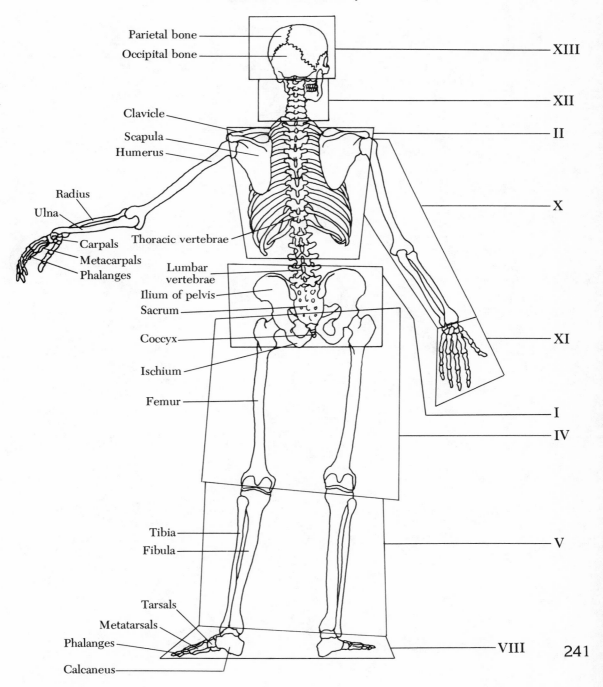

Parietal bone

Occipital bone

XIII

XII

II

Clavicle

Scapula

Humerus

X

Radius

Ulna

Thoracic vertebrae

Carpals

Metacarpals

Phalanges

Lumbar vertebrae

Ilium of pelvis

Sacrum

Coccyx

XI

Ischium

Femur

I

IV

Tibia

Fibula

V

Tarsals

Metatarsals

Phalanges

VIII

Calcaneus

241

PLATE 3
MUSCLE MAN, FRONT VIEW

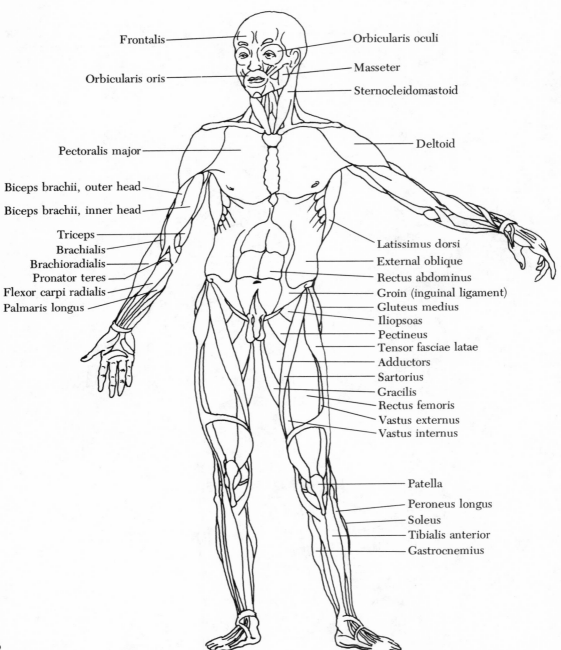

Frontalis

Orbicularis oris

Pectoralis major

Biceps brachii, outer head

Biceps brachii, inner head

Triceps

Brachialis

Brachioradialis

Pronator teres

Flexor carpi radialis

Palmaris longus

Orbicularis oculi

Masseter

Sternocleidomastoid

Deltoid

Latissimus dorsi

External oblique

Rectus abdominus

Groin (inguinal ligament)

Gluteus medius

Iliopsoas

Pectineus

Tensor fasciae latae

Adductors

Sartorius

Gracilis

Rectus femoris

Vastus externus

Vastus internus

Patella

Peroneus longus

Soleus

Tibialis anterior

Gastrocnemius

PLATE 4
MUSCLE MAN, BACK VIEW

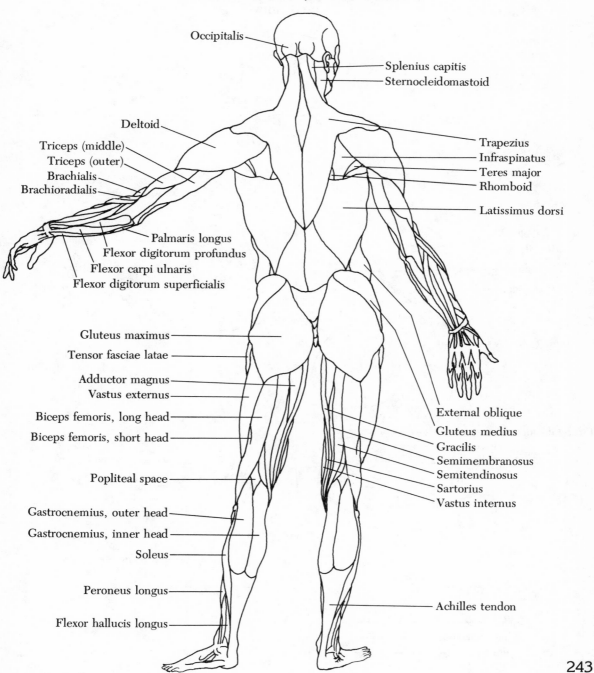

Occipitalis

Splenius capitis

Sternocleidomastoid

Deltoid

Triceps (middle)

Triceps (outer)

Brachialis

Brachioradialis

Trapezius

Infraspinatus

Teres major

Rhomboid

Latissimus dorsi

Palmaris longus

Flexor digitorum profundus

Flexor carpi ulnaris

Flexor digitorum superficialis

Gluteus maximus

Tensor fasciae latae

Adductor magnus

Vastus externus

Biceps femoris, long head

Biceps femoris, short head

External oblique

Gluteus medius

Gracilis

Semimembranosus

Semitendinosus

Sartorius

Vastus internus

Popliteal space

Gastrocnemius, outer head

Gastrocnemius, inner head

Soleus

Peroneus longus

Flexor hallucis longus

Achilles tendon

243

PLATE 5

THE TORSO, BACK VIEW
Sections I and II

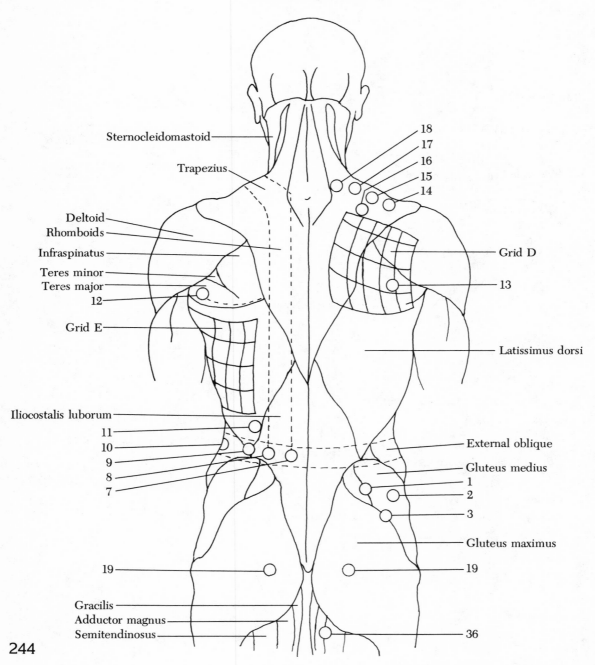

Sternocleidomastoid

18
17
16
15
14

Trapezius

Deltoid
Rhomboids
Infraspinatus

Grid D

Teres minor
Teres major
12

13

Grid E

Iliocostalis luborum

Latissimus dorsi

11
10
9
8
7

External oblique

Gluteus medius

1
2
3

Gluteus maximus

19

19

Gracilis
Adductor magnus
Semitendinosus

36

PLATE 6

THE TORSO, FRONT VIEW
Sections III, IX, XII, XV

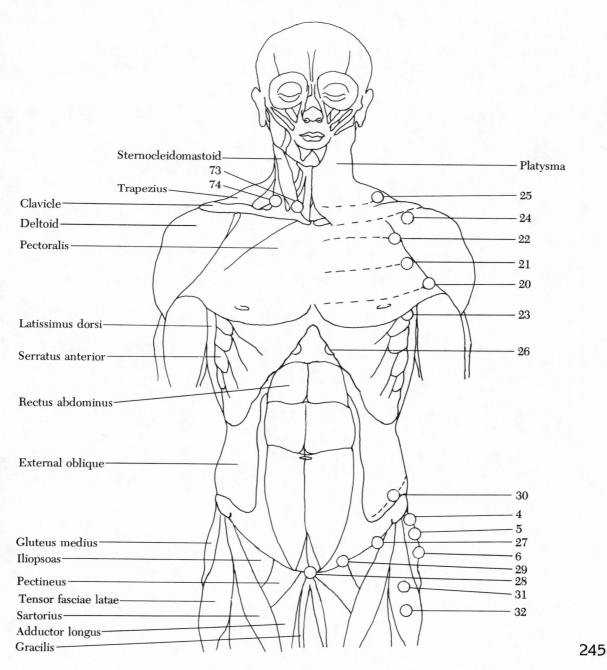

Sternocleidomastoid
73
74
Trapezius
Clavicle
Deltoid
Pectoralis

Latissimus dorsi
Serratus anterior

Rectus abdominus

External oblique

Gluteus medius
Iliopsoas
Pectineus
Tensor fasciae latae
Sartorius
Adductor longus
Gracilis

Platysma
25
24
22
21
20
23
26
30
4
5
27
6
29
28
31
32

PLATE 7

THE LEG, FRONT VIEW
Sections VI and VII

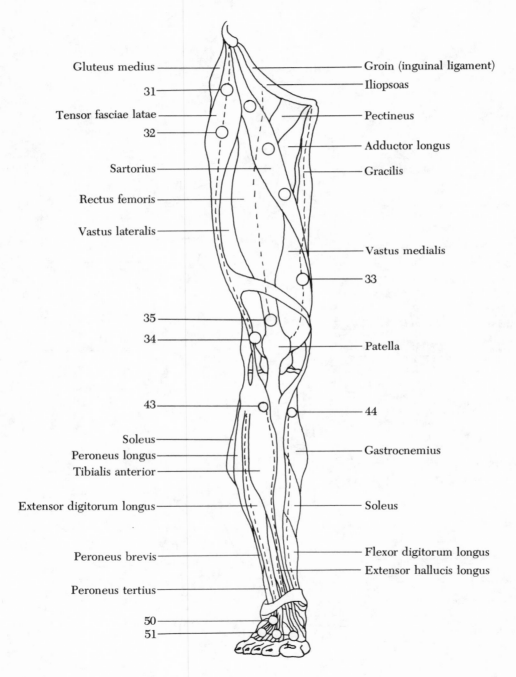

Gluteus medius

31

Tensor fasciae latae

32

Sartorius

Rectus femoris

Vastus lateralis

35

34

43

Soleus

Peroneus longus

Tibialis anterior

Extensor digitorum longus

Peroneus brevis

Peroneus tertius

50
51

Groin (inguinal ligament)

Iliopsoas

Pectineus

Adductor longus

Gracilis

Vastus medialis

33

Patella

44

Gastrocnemius

Soleus

Flexor digitorum longus

Extensor hallucis longus

PLATE 8

THE LEG, BACK VIEW
Sections IV and V

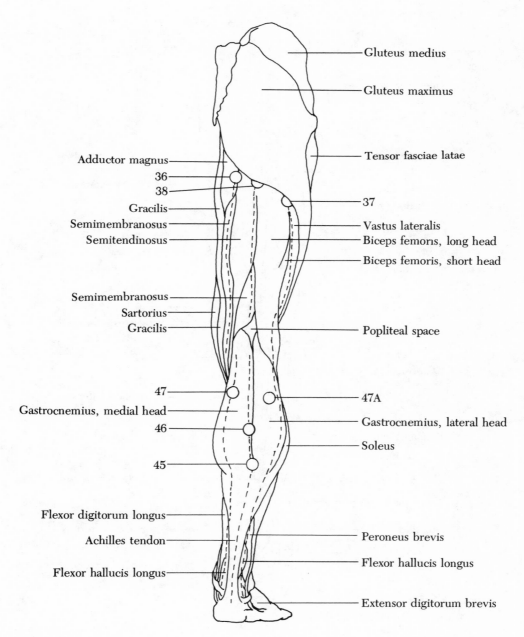

Gluteus medius

Gluteus maximus

Tensor fasciae latae

Adductor magnus
36
38
Gracilis
Semimembranosus
Semitendinosus

37
Vastus lateralis
Biceps femoris, long head
Biceps femoris, short head

Semimembranosus
Sartorius
Gracilis

Popliteal space

47
Gastrocnemius, medial head
46
45

47A
Gastrocnemius, lateral head
Soleus

Flexor digitorum longus
Achilles tendon

Peroneus brevis
Flexor hallucis longus

Flexor hallucis longus

Extensor digitorum brevis

PLATE 9

THE LEG, OUTSIDE VIEW
Sections IV through VII

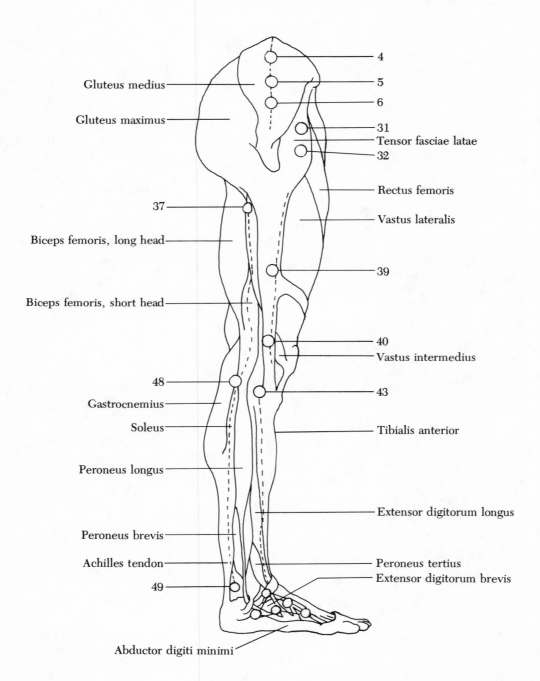

Gluteus medius

Gluteus maximus

4

5

6

31

Tensor fasciae latae

32

Rectus femoris

Vastus lateralis

37

Biceps femoris, long head

39

Biceps femoris, short head

40

Vastus intermedius

48

43

Gastrocnemius

Soleus

Tibialis anterior

Peroneus longus

Extensor digitorum longus

Peroneus brevis

Achilles tendon

Peroneus tertius

Extensor digitorum brevis

49

Abductor digiti minimi

PLATE 10

THE LEG, INSIDE VIEW
Sections IV through VII

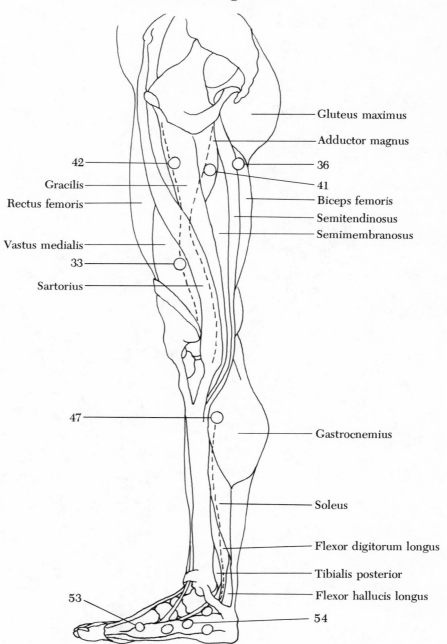

Gluteus maximus

Adductor magnus

42

Gracilis

Rectus femoris

36

41

Biceps femoris

Semitendinosus

Semimembranosus

Vastus medialis

33

Sartorius

47

Gastrocnemius

Soleus

Flexor digitorum longus

Tibialis posterior

Flexor hallucis longus

53

54

PLATE 11
THE FOOT
Section VIII

Dorsal View

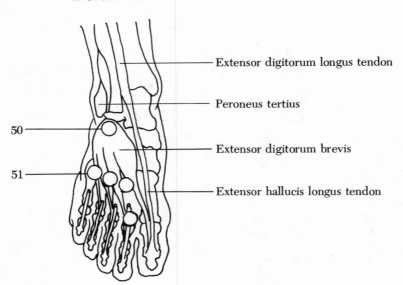

— Extensor digitorum longus tendon

— Peroneus tertius

50 —

— Extensor digitorum brevis

51 —

— Extensor hallucis longus tendon

Plantar View (Sole)

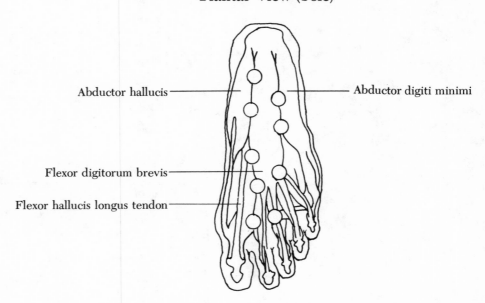

Abductor hallucis —

— Abductor digiti minimi

Flexor digitorum brevis —

Flexor hallucis longus tendon —

PLATE 12

FRONT OF HEAD AND FACE
Sections XIII and XIV

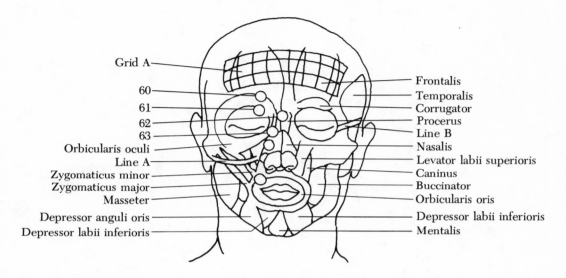

Grid A

60
61
62
63
Orbicularis oculi
Line A
Zygomaticus minor
Zygomaticus major
Masseter
Depressor anguli oris
Depressor labii inferioris

Frontalis
Temporalis
Corrugator
Procerus
Line B
Nasalis
Levator labii superioris
Caninus
Buccinator
Orbicularis oris
Depressor labii inferioris
Mentalis

PLATE 13

BACK OF HEAD, NECK, AND UPPER BACK
Sections II, XII, and XIII

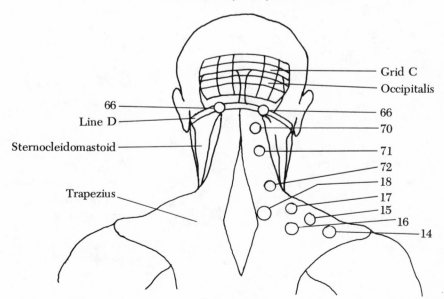

66
Line D
Sternocleidomastoid

Trapezius

Grid C
Occipitalis
66
70
71
72
18
17
15
16
14

251

PLATE 14

THE NECK
Sections XII and XIII

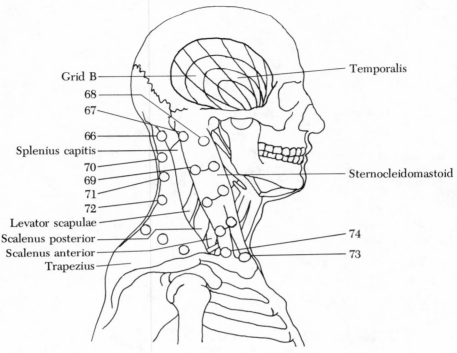

Grid B

68

67

66

Splenius capitis

70

69

71

72

Levator scapulae

Scalenus posterior

Scalenus anterior

Trapezius

Temporalis

Sternocleidomastoid

74

73

PLATE 15

THE SIDE OF HEAD, FACE, AND NECK
Sections XII, XIII, and XIV

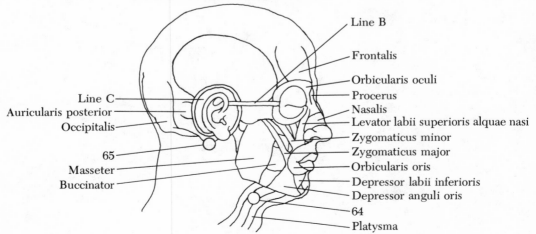

Line C

Auricularis posterior

Occipitalis

65

Masseter

Buccinator

Line B

Frontalis

Orbicularis oculi

Procerus

Nasalis

Levator labii superioris alquae nasi

Zygomaticus minor

Zygomaticus major

Orbicularis oris

Depressor labii inferioris

Depressor anguli oris

64

Platysma

252

PLATE 16

THE ANTERIOR ARM (Pronated)
Sections X and XI

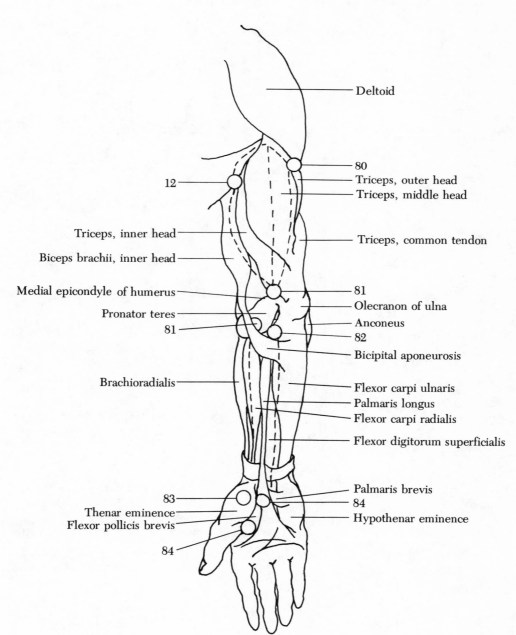

Deltoid

80
Triceps, outer head
Triceps, middle head

12

Triceps, inner head

Triceps, common tendon

Biceps brachii, inner head

Medial epicondyle of humerus

81
Olecranon of ulna

Pronator teres

Anconeus

81

82

Bicipital aponeurosis

Brachioradialis

Flexor carpi ulnaris
Palmaris longus
Flexor carpi radialis

Flexor digitorum superficialis

Palmaris brevis

83

84

Thenar eminence

Hypothenar eminence

Flexor pollicis brevis

84

PLATE 17

THE POSTERIOR ARM (Pronated)
Sections X and XI

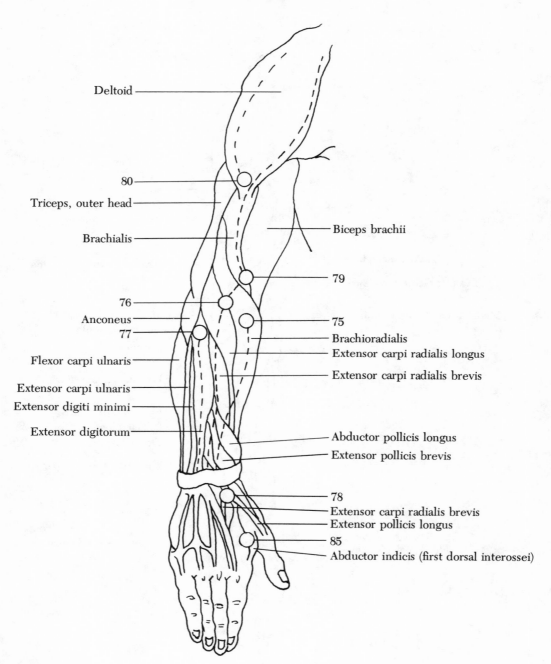

Deltoid

80

Triceps, outer head

Brachialis

Biceps brachii

79

76

75

Anconeus

77

Brachioradialis

Extensor carpi radialis longus

Flexor carpi ulnaris

Extensor carpi radialis brevis

Extensor carpi ulnaris

Extensor digiti minimi

Extensor digitorum

Abductor pollicis longus

Extensor pollicis brevis

78

Extensor carpi radialis brevis

Extensor pollicis longus

85

Abductor indicis (first dorsal interossei)

PLATE 18

THE AXILLA
Section XVI

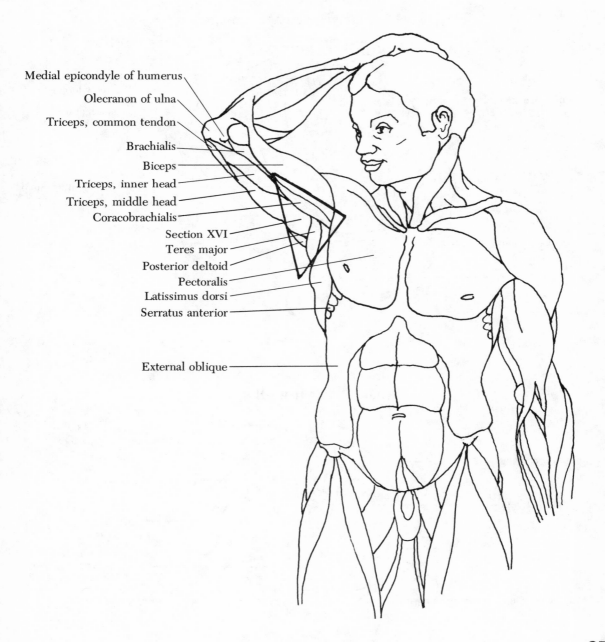

Medial epicondyle of humerus

Olecranon of ulna

Triceps, common tendon

Brachialis

Biceps

Triceps, inner head

Triceps, middle head

Coracobrachialis

Section XVI

Teres major

Posterior deltoid

Pectoralis

Latissimus dorsi

Serratus anterior

External oblique

PLATE 19

THE PELVIC FLOOR (Levator Ani)
Section XVII

Male Pelvis from Above

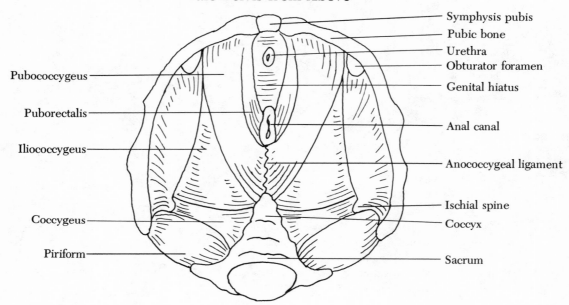

Pubococcygeus

Puborectalis

Iliococcygeus

Coccygeus

Piriform

Symphysis pubis
Pubic bone
Urethra
Obturator foramen
Genital hiatus

Anal canal

Anococcygeal ligament

Ischial spine
Coccyx

Sacrum

Female Pelvis from Below

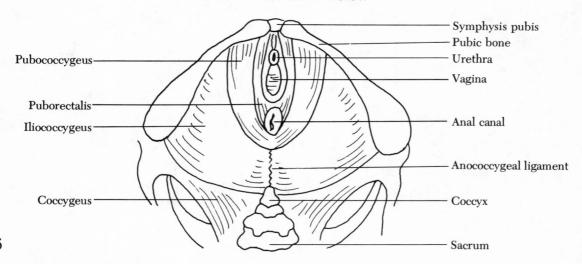

Pubococcygeus

Puborectalis
Iliococcygeus

Coccygeus

Symphysis pubis
Pubic bone
Urethra
Vagina

Anal canal

Anococcygeal ligament

Coccyx

Sacrum

Appendix 2

Table of Pains and Other Symptoms, Giving Areas of the Body Harboring Related Trigger Points

The roman numerals in the table refer to the areas of the body as described in Appendix 1. The body areas listed for each pain or symptom should be cleared of trigger points in the order given. Techniques for clearing trigger points are explained in appropriate chapters throughout the book.

Be sure that before you begin your hunt for the cause of chronic pain you consult a physician or dentist to ascertain that the condition is muscular and there is no anatomic pathology.

Kind of Pain or Symptom	Body Areas
Ankle pain	III, VI, IV, V, VII, VIII
Arm pain	X, IX, II, XI
Back, lower	I, II, III, IV
Back, mid	II, I, III, IX
Back, upper	II, I, IX, III, XII, X
Bursitis (shoulder)	X, IX, II, XII, XI, XVI
Carpal tunnel syndrome	X, XI, II, IX, XVI

Kind of Pain or Symptom	Body Areas
Chest pain	IX, II, X, XI, XII, XVI
Circulation, poor, and cold feet	VI, IV, III, V, VIII
Cramps, abdominal	III, XV, I, IV, VI
Cramps, legs	V, IV, I, VII, VI, III, VIII
Cramps, menstrual	III, XV, I, IV
Disc problems	I, II, III, IV
Dizziness	XIV, VIII, XII, IX, II
Double vision	XIV, XIII, XII
Duck walk (turned-out feet)	I, VI, IV, V, VII, VIII
Earache	XIII, XIV, XII
Fracture (see page 260)	
Frigidity	I, III
Frozen shoulder (stiff)	IX, II, X, XI, XII
Groin pain	III, I, IV, VI
Growing pains	I, III, IV, VI, V, VII, VIII
Hangover	XIII, XIV, XII
Headache	XIV, XIII, XII, IX, II, X
Hemorrhoids	I, III
Hip pain	I, III, IV, VI, XV, II
Impotence	I, III
Knee pain	VI, V, IV, VIII, III, I
Kyphosis (extreme round back)	IX, X, II, XV, III
Long second toe	VII, V, VIII, VI, IV
Neck pain	II, XII, XIII, IX, X
Numb fingers	IX, II, X, XVI, XI
Osgood-Schlatter disease	VI, V, IV, VIII, III, I
Phantom limb pain (arm)	IX, II, XVI, XII (work back to stump and do stump as well) *Do other arm.*
Phantom limb pain (leg)	III, I, XV (work back to stump and do stump as well) *Do other leg.*
Pigeon toes (turned-in feet)	I, IV, VI, V, VII
Pregnancy	I, III, XV, IV, VI, V, VII
Scars (See page 260)	
Sciatica	I, IV
Scoliosis (spinal curvature)	I, II, XV, III, IV
Shinsplints	I, III, IV, V, VI, VII

Kind of Pain or Symptom	*Body Areas*
Shoulder pain	IX, II, X, XI, XII
Sinus pain	XIV, XIII, XII
Stitches (pains in side from running)	III, XV, I
Stroke, arm	X, XI, IX, II
Stroke, leg	I, II, III, IV, V, VI, VII
Swelling in the legs	I, III, IV, V, VI, VII, VIII
Temporomandibular joint dysfunction (jaw pain)	XIV, XIII, XII, IX, II, X, XI
Tennis elbow	X, XI, IX, II
Tic douloureux	XIV, XIII, XII
Tingling fingers	II, IX, X, XI
Tinnitis (ringing in ears)	XIII, XIV, XII, II
Toothache	XII, XIV, XIII
Torticollis (neck tightness)	XIII, XIV, XII, IX, II, X
Varicose veins	I, III, IV, VI, V, VII, VIII
Whiplash	XIII, XIV, XII, IX, II, X
Wrist	II, IX, X, XI

Loss of balance, poor coordination, and weakness, all are often caused by trigger points in the legs. Get rid of them.

Diseases such as rheumatoid arthritis, lupus, multiple sclerosis, Parkinson's, psoriatic arthritis, as well as conditions such as cerebral palsy and brain damage, lay down patterns of muscle spasm and pain. These diseases do not have specific patterns of trigger points, but myotherapy can help most of the time. Just seek out the area suffering pain and check with the plates for the most likely offenders.

There can be muscle contraction without pain as in cerebral palsy. This also responds to myotherapy.

When the disease is one that attacks in cycles—MS, rheumatoid, and lupus, for example—the trigger points can be erased to give relief, but when the disease flares again the pain will return. The trigger points must be erased again. Conditions in which joints are diseased will cause almost continuous pain. The trigger points then must be erased on a continuing basis.

Pain of long standing (such as migraines) may need two to three months of trigger point work before the pain is permanently controlled. Recurrence of pain usually means some trigger points were overlooked.

Trigger points are often housed in the muscles surrounding any scar tissue resulting from wounds, either accidents or operations. This is true also of healed fractures. Clear the entire section where the fracture or scar is.

Appendix 3
Table of Occupations and Related Pain Hazards

OCCUPATIONS CLASSIFIED BY KIND OR DEGREE OF PHYSICAL ACTIVITY REQUIRED

Sitting	Standing	Walking	Active	Strenuous
Accountant	Bank teller	Detective	Carpenter	Athlete
Administrator	Barber	Flight attendant	Carpet layer	Construction worker
Anesthetist	Bartender	Floorwalker	Dairy worker	Dancer
Architect	Beautician	Librarian	Electrician	Diver
Artist	Blacksmith	Nurse	Farmer	Heavy equipment
Astronaut	Butcher	Orderly	Farrier	operator
Author	Cafeteria server	Postman	Fireman	Linesman
Bookkeeper	Clerk	Real estate agent	Forester	Longshoreman
Broadcaster	Cook	Service station	Groom	Martial arts
Bus driver	Dental hygienist	attendant	Maintenance	instructor
Cabbie	Dentist	Train conductor	Mason	Masseur and
Chauffeur	Doctor	Usher	Mechanic	masseuse
Computer programmer	Electrologist	Waitress	Painter	Miner
Crane operator	Elevator operator	Watchman	Photographer	Steelworker
Dispatcher	File clerk		Plumber	Woodsman
Draftsman	Hairdresser		Policeman	
Editor	Machinist		Sailor	
Educator	Salesclerk		Ski instructor	
Electronics repairer	Sculptor		Soldier	
Engineer	Surgeon		Sports coach	
Executive	Veterinarian		Tree man	
Glass blower				
Jeweler				
Keypunch operator				
Lawyer				
Pilot				
Psychiatrist				
School bus driver				
Secretary				
Student				
Teacher				
Telephone operator				
Trucker				
Weaver				

RELATED PAIN HAZARDS

Sitting

Sitting occupations often put trigger points in the upper and lower back (sections I and II). Since the body is constantly bent, the groin (III) may well be involved. If circulation is impaired by overweight, the legs and buttocks, which are constantly compressed against chairs, will become involved (sections IV, V, VI, VII).

Standing

Occupations requiring long hours of standing in one place contribute to the risk of low back pain (I). The upper back (II) too is endangered, as are the arms (X) and the shoulders and neck (XII). There may also be swelling in the feet and ankles (VIII, VII, and V).

Walking

Occupations requiring ordinary walking are not at risk. However, when the walking includes carrying (postman or waitress) the back (I and II) is in danger.

Active

Active occupations all entail dangers. For example, carpenters damage their elbows and suffer from "tennis elbow," the plumber working with pipe threaders and large wrenches puts trigger points in his chest muscles. The mason strains his back. The dancer damages his legs and lower back.

Strenuous

Strenuous occupations all too often result in back pain, and the injuries often involve torque—the ladder that gets away, the barrel that rolls wrong—anything that pulls the torso with a twisting motion.

Whatever the occupation, if the work being done by the hands and arms is repetitious the arms (X), chest (IX), and upper back (II) may feel stiffness or pain. Musicians holding their instruments in one position, and dentists, too, may house trigger points in the upper back (II) and neck (XII).

If the back is constantly rounded by requirements of the job, the pain may appear in the upper back (II). The pulling from shortened pectoral muscles should also be investigated (IX).

Housework has many perils, but the usual complaint is back pain. Pregnancy, while not an occupation, deserves comment since it often causes backache and leg and foot pain as well as leg swelling.

Note your category and prepare against pain by keeping the area at risk clear of trigger points. Don't forget to build resistance with the exercises you need.

Appendix 4

Table of Sports and Related Pain Hazards

Here is a list of the major sports. For each sport certain parts of the body come under stress. You will find those vulnerable sections listed after each sport. To *prevent* injury, clear these areas systematically *before* and *after* the game with seeking massage (see Chapter 7). Erase from the sections in the order given.

Keep track of the improvement in your performance and note which muscles were worked before that trial. Any muscles in tonic spasm that interfere with your performance will be found by this method.

Sports	*Body Sections Under Stress*
Archery	IX, II, X, XII, XVI
Badminton	Same as Tennis
Baseball	I, II, III, XV, X, XI, V, XVI
Basketball	I, II, III, XV, XVI, IX, IV, V, VI, VII
Bike riding	I, II, IV, V, VI, VII, III
Bird-watching	XII, II, IX, IV, VI, V, VII
Bowling	I, II, IX, X, VI
Boxing	IX, X, II, XVI
Camping	According to individual weakness
Canoeing	IX, II, X, XV, III, XVI
Cross country running	IV, VI, V, VII, III, XV, I
Cross country skiing	IX, X, II, I, XVI, IV, V, VI, VII
Dancing, ballet	IV, V, VI, VII, VIII, III, XV, I
Dancing, ballroom	Pretty safe
Dancing, modern	Same as Ballet Dancing
Diving	X, II, IX

Sports	*Body Sections Under Stress*
Field hockey	IV, V, VI, VII, III, XV, I
Figure skating	IV, V, VI, VII, III, XI, II, IX
Fishing (deep sea)	II, I, X, IX, IV, V, VI, VII, XVI
Fishing (stream)	IV, V, VI, VII, I, II, X
Football	Everything
Gardening	I, II, III, X, XI
Golf	I, II, XV, III, IX
Gymnastics	Everything
Handball	IV, V, VI, VII, I, II, IX, X, XI
Hiking	IV, V, VI, VII, I, II
Hunting	Same as Hiking
Ice hockey	Everything
Lacrosse	Everything
Marathon running	IV, V, VI, VII, I, II, III, XV
Mountaineering	IV, V, VI, VII, XV, I, II, IX
Paddle tennis	Same as Tennis
Racquet ball	Same as Tennis
Riding	VI, IV, II, X, IX, XV, III
Rock climbing	IV, V, VI, VII, X, XI, XV
Rowing	II, IX, X, IV, V, VI, VII, I
Running	IV, V, VI, VII, III, XV, I
Sailing	X, II, IX, XVI
Scuba diving	I, III
Skiing, downhill	IV, V, VI, VII, III, I
Slalom	Same as Downhill Skiing
Soccer	Everything
Sports cars	X, IX, II
Squash	Same as Tennis
Swim, competition (back stroke)	X, IX, II, XVI
Swim, competition (breast stroke)	IX, X, XVI, XV, III
Swim, competition (crawl)	X, IX, II, III, IV, VI, XV, XVI
Swimming for fun	Pretty safe
Tennis	IV, V, VI, VII, VIII, III, I, II, XV, IX, X, XVI
Track	IV, V, VI, VII, III, I, XV
Volleyball	IV, V, VI, VII, IX, X, XVI
Water skiing	IV, V, VI, VII, III, X, XVI, XV, II
White-water canoeing	IX, II, X, XV, XVI
Wrestling	Everything

265

Sources

BOOKS

Crile, George, Jr. *Surgery: Your Choices and Your Alternatives.* New York: Delacorte Press, 1978.
If you think you need surgery, be aware that there are almost always alternatives. This book is a good guide to them.

Leboyer, Frederick. *Loving Hands.* New York: Alfred A. Knopf, 1976.
A very complete guide to baby massage.

———. *Birth Without Violence.* New York: Alfred A. Knopf, 1975.
A guide to less frightening birthdays for babies.

Montagu, Ashley. *Touching.* New York: Perennial Library, 1972.
The skin regarded as a sense organ.

Prudden, Bonnie. *Bonnie Prudden's Fitness Book.* New York: Ronald Press, 1959.
Personalized exercise programs. Indoor and outdoor exercise equipment.

———. *How to Keep Slender and Fit After Thirty.* Rev. ed. New York: Bernard Geis Associates, 1966, and New York: Pocket Books, 1970.
A complete exercise program plus the philosophy needed to implement it after age thirty.

———. *How to Keep Your Child Fit from Birth to Six.* New York: Harper and Row, Publishers, 1964.
Exercises should begin at birth since the major damage resulting from sedentary living is visited on children *before* school days. Parents can prevent it by providing appropriate physical activity from babyhood on.

———. *Fitness from Six to Twelve.* New York: Harper and Row, Publishers, 1972.
American schools are not equipped to repair the physical and emotional damage resulting from years of exposure to sedentary TV viewing and confinement to strollers, car seats, high chairs, and playpens. The second six years of life make up the last block of time in which to build a good

body for a child. This book is a complete guide for parents who want to build such bodies for both boys and girls.

———. *Teenage Fitness.* New York: Harper and Row, Publishers, 1965.

People are now aware that physical fitness is a necessity, and Title IX has given the green light to athletics for girls equal to that for boys. Unfortunately, few know how to start or what to do. A good coed program of physical activity for young people as well as the philosophy needed for implementation. Pre-sport conditioning and how-to exercises.

———. *Your Baby Can Swim.* Stockbridge, Mass: Aquarian Press, 1977.

How to teach your baby to become water-wise.

———.*How to Keep Your Family Fit and Healthy.* Stockbridge, Mass.: Aquarian Press, 1977.

Families want to exercise together, but what programs appeal to every age and can be adapted for each generation? This book has that information.

———. *Ever-Sex.* Stockbridge, Mass.: Aquarian Press, 1979.

A gentle book about feelings and sex, with exercises that improve both as well as the quality of life. A different, better way of imparting information about sex and loving.

———. *Physical Fitness For You (A Talking Book for the Blind).* New York: American Foundation for the Blind, 1964.

The complete book of exercise for the blind, partially blind and older people who may be limited in their exercise programs by age or handicaps. It can be ordered from The American Foundation for the Blind at 15 West 16 Street, New York, New York 10011.

VIDEOS

Prudden, Bonnie. *Keep Fit . . . Be Happy, Volume I.* Los Angeles: Warner Brothers, 1959.

An excellent starting program of exercise with delightful music. A special aerobics band for running at home and two bands on progressive relaxation.

———. *Keep Fit . . . Be Happy, Volume II.* Los Angeles: Warner Brothers, 1961.

Advanced exercise plus floor progressions, weight lifting, and a tumbling routine.

EQUIPMENT

If you have read this book you know that Bodos are handmade wooden tools used for erasing muscle pain by extinguishing trigger points. One of their chief values is they can be used by people who don't have live-in exercise therapists or myotherapists but must depend on their own hands. Available only from Bonnie Prudden, 800–221–4634.

MYOTHERAPY HELP LINE

For information, mail order catalog, myotherapy and exercise videos, tapes, books, self-help tools, equipment, annual brochure, gift certificates, clothing, trigger point charts, weekend seminars, career training, pain-free living workshops, Bonnie Prudden School and Certification Program, Directory of Certified Bonnie Prudden Myotherapists call 800-221-4634.

Index

269

ABOUT THE AUTHOR

BONNIE PRUDDEN has been one of the world's leading authorities on physical fitness and exercise therapy for over two decades. Her research on the fitness of American children helped create the President's Council on Physical Fitness and Sports in the 1950s. Director of the Institute for Physical Fitness and Myotherapy in Stockbridge, Massachusetts, Mrs. Prudden has written numerous books and articles on exercise and health.